Psychiatric Prescribing Quick Reference

A Diagnosis-Based Clinical Guide to Psychopharmacology for PMHNPs and Advanced Practice Providers

Conor Gino Pettersson

This book is intended for use as an educational and clinical reference tool for licensed healthcare professionals, including psychiatric mental health nurse practitioners, physician assistants, physicians, and other qualified prescribers. The information provided reflects evidence-based clinical practice as of the date of publication and is not a substitute for professional clinical judgment, individualized patient assessment, or consultation with specialists when clinically indicated. Medication dosing, indications, contraindications, and monitoring recommendations may change as new evidence emerges, FDA labeling is updated, and clinical guidelines are revised. Prescribers are responsible for verifying current prescribing information, checking for drug interactions, and confirming appropriateness for each individual patient before initiating, modifying, or discontinuing any medication discussed in this book.

All clinical case examples presented in this book are fictional composites created for educational purposes. Names, demographic details, clinical histories, and treatment scenarios are entirely fabricated and do not represent any actual patient, living or deceased. Any resemblance to real individuals is purely coincidental. These examples are designed to illustrate clinical concepts and prescribing principles and should not be interpreted as specific treatment recommendations for any individual patient.

The publisher and copyright holder assume no liability for errors, omissions, or outcomes resulting from the use of information

First Edition, 2026

978-1-7645863-1-3

Table of Contents

Preface

The fifteen-minute medication management visit is not enough time. Every prescriber who has ever watched the clock while simultaneously confirming a diagnosis, reviewing labs, assessing suicide risk, managing a drug interaction question, and trying to make a thoughtful prescribing decision knows that fifteen minutes is not enough. And yet, it is what most clinical schedules provide. The question, then, is not how to get more time. The question is how to use those fifteen minutes with maximum clinical precision.

Psychiatric prescribing has grown more complex in the past five years than in the preceding twenty. The 2024 and 2025 FDA approval cycles brought the first non-dopaminergic antipsychotic mechanism in decades, monotherapy options for treatment-resistant depression that previously required combination regimens, expanded indications for atypical antipsychotics across mood disorders, and regulatory changes that simultaneously improved access to clozapine and tightened benzodiazepine prescribing guidance. Pharmacogenomic testing has moved from academic curiosity to clinical utility, with CPIC guidelines now covering more than twenty-five psychiatric medications. Practice guidelines from the APA, VA/DoD, CANMAT, and ten-society collaborations have reshaped the evidence base for conditions from PTSD to insomnia to bipolar maintenance.

The existing references have not kept pace with how prescribers actually need to access this information. Drug-class-organized textbooks require the prescriber to already know which medication class is appropriate before looking anything up. That is exactly backward from clinical reality, where the patient presents with a symptom cluster and the prescriber needs to determine the best pharmacological approach. General prescribing references that cover all medical diagnoses devote only a fraction of their content to psychiatric medications, leaving advanced psychiatric prescribers without the depth they require. And the pocketbook guides that promise simplicity sacrifice the clinical nuance that distinguishes competent prescribing from reflexive prescribing.

This reference was designed to close that gap. The organizing principle is the clinical encounter itself. A patient presents with a complaint. The prescriber confirms a diagnosis. A decision tree guides medication selection based on the patient's specific symptom profile, medical comorbidities, reproductive status, pharmacogenomic data, and treatment history. Monitoring parameters are embedded at every prescribing decision point, not isolated in a separate chapter. Augmentation strategies, treatment-resistant pathways, and medication switching protocols follow the same branching logic that clinical decision-making demands.

The twenty-six chapters and six appendices that follow are structured to serve two modes of use. The first is real-time clinical reference: a prescriber with a patient in front of them, a specific question, and limited time. The decision trees, dosing tables, interaction references, and monitoring checklists are designed for this speed. The second mode is clinical education: a student, resident, or early-career prescriber building the pharmacological knowledge base that supports confident, independent practice. The chapter narratives, case examples, and evidence summaries serve this deeper learning.

Throughout the book, the neuroscience is clinical, not academic. Receptor pharmacology is presented as the basis for predicting therapeutic effects and side effects, not as abstract biology. Pharmacokinetics are translated into practical prescribing decisions about drug interactions, switching protocols, and dose adjustments. Pharmacogenomics are applied, with specific guidance on when to test, how to interpret results, and what to do with the information. Special populations (perinatal, pediatric, geriatric, medically complex) receive dedicated chapters because the prescribing adjustments these patients require are not footnotes. They are distinct clinical skill sets.

The field of psychopharmacology will continue to evolve. New medications will receive approval. Guidelines will be updated. Evidence will shift prescribing recommendations. But the clinical logic of this book, moving from patient presentation through diagnostic confirmation to evidence-based medication selection with embedded monitoring, will remain sound regardless of which specific medications occupy the decision tree nodes. That architecture is the enduring contribution this reference offers to the prescribers who use it daily.

The fifteen-minute visit is not enough time to figure it out from scratch. It is enough time to look it up, confirm the plan, and prescribe with confidence. That is what these pages are for.

How to Use This Book

You are holding a clinical tool, not a textbook you read cover to cover. This book was designed for one purpose: to get you from a patient's presenting complaint to an evidence-based prescribing decision as fast as possible. Every page, every decision tree, every monitoring parameter exists because a busy prescriber in a 15-minute medication management appointment needs the answer now.

Organized by Presentation

Most psychopharmacology references organize content by drug class. Antidepressants in one section, antipsychotics in another, mood stabilizers somewhere else. That structure makes sense for pharmacology courses. It does not make sense when a patient is sitting across from you describing persistent sadness, poor sleep, and anhedonia, and you need to determine the best medication strategy for their specific presentation.

This book is organized by diagnosis and clinical presentation. When your patient presents with treatment-resistant depression, you turn to Chapter 5.0 and find a decision tree that walks you through augmentation strategies, switching protocols, and esketamine considerations. When a patient with schizophrenia develops tardive dyskinesia on their current antipsychotic, Chapter 10.0 gives you the VMAT2 inhibitor comparison and side effect management pathway. The clinical question drives the structure. Always.

Each diagnosis-based chapter follows the same internal architecture. You will find diagnostic confirmation criteria first, followed by first-line medication selection organized as a decision tree. Second-line and augmentation strategies come next, with clear branching logic for partial response versus nonresponse. Monitoring parameters are embedded at every decision point, not relegated to an appendix you have to flip to separately. Special population considerations (pregnancy, pediatric, geriatric, hepatic or renal impairment) are flagged with icons throughout the text rather than siloed into separate chapters you might forget to check.

Decision Tree Architecture

The decision trees in this book are not decorative. They are the spine of your clinical workflow. Each tree begins with the confirmed diagnosis, moves through first-line medication selection based on symptom cluster and patient factors, and then branches according to treatment response at defined time intervals. For major depressive disorder, the tree asks: Has the patient achieved at least 50% symptom reduction at 4 weeks? If yes, optimize and continue. If no, the tree branches into switching versus augmentation pathways, each with specific medication recommendations, dosing parameters, and monitoring requirements.

Decision points are marked with the clinical question that triggers the branch. "Is the patient tolerating the current medication?" leads one direction. "Has the patient failed two adequate antidepressant trials?" leads to the treatment-resistant depression pathway with esketamine, MAOIs, and somatic treatment considerations. You follow the logic from where your patient is right now to where you need to go next.

Icons and Formatting Legend

Throughout this book, you will encounter standardized icons that flag critical prescribing information at a glance:

- **[BBW]** Black Box Warning. The FDA's highest safety alert. Stop and read before prescribing.
- **[OL]** Off-Label Use. The medication is being recommended for an indication not included in the FDA-approved labeling. Evidence level is noted.

- **[PG]** Pharmacogenomic Alert. CYP450 metabolism or HLA screening may affect dosing or drug selection. Cross-reference Chapter 3.0 for interpretation guidance.
- **[PREG]** Pregnancy Consideration. Reproductive safety data exists that may influence prescribing. Cross-reference Chapter 18.0 for detailed perinatal guidance.
- **[$]** Cost Alert. Significant price differential exists between options. Generic availability and patient assistance programs noted where relevant.
- **[MON]** Monitoring Required. Specific laboratory, vital sign, or clinical monitoring is required at baseline or during treatment.
- **[NEW]** Newly Approved. Medication or indication received FDA approval in 2024 or 2025. Evidence base and clinical positioning are current as of publication.

These icons appear inline with the text, immediately adjacent to the medication or recommendation they modify. You do not need to flip to a separate legend page after the first reading. They become intuitive within the first chapter you use clinically.

Cross-Referencing System

Psychiatric patients rarely present with a single, uncomplicated diagnosis. The patient with major depressive disorder also has generalized anxiety. The patient with ADHD has a comorbid substance use disorder. The patient with bipolar disorder is pregnant. This book anticipates those intersections.

Cross-references appear as bracketed callouts throughout each chapter. When a decision tree for depression reaches the branch point where bipolar features need to be ruled out, you will see: *See section 6.1 for bipolar screening and diagnostic clarification.* When a patient with schizophrenia requires clozapine and has hepatic impairment, the text directs you to *section 21.1 for hepatic adjustment guidelines.* These cross-references use the section numbering system consistently. You will always know exactly where to find the related content.

Comorbidity tables at the end of each diagnosis-based chapter summarize the most common co-occurring conditions and point you to the relevant sections. If you are managing PTSD and the patient also has alcohol use disorder, the comorbidity table in Chapter 9.0 directs you to section 13.1 for integrated medication approaches.

Quick-Flip Tab Structure

The physical layout of this book is designed for speed. Part II (Chapters 5 through 17) contains the diagnosis-based prescribing guides that will constitute 80% of your daily use. These chapters are organized with thumb tabs along the edge for rapid access. Part IV (Chapters 23 through 26) contains the reference tables, algorithms, and monitoring schedules you will pull from repeatedly during clinical sessions.

For a typical 15-minute medication management appointment, your workflow might look like this: Patient presents with worsening anxiety despite six weeks of sertraline 100mg. You flip to Chapter 7.0 (Anxiety Disorders), locate the GAD decision tree, and follow the partial-response branch. The tree suggests dose optimization to 150-200mg or augmentation with buspirone. Monitoring parameters are listed at that decision node. You check the CYP450 interaction flag because the patient takes omeprazole. You reference the pharmacogenomic alert because a previous trial of citalopram produced intolerable side effects. The cross-reference directs you to section 3.2 for CYP2C19 considerations. Total time to informed decision: under three minutes.

That is how this book is meant to work. Not as reading material. As a clinical instrument.

A Note on Evidence Levels

Medication recommendations throughout this book are graded according to the strength of supporting evidence. Level A recommendations are supported by multiple randomized controlled trials or meta-analyses. Level B recommendations are supported by a single randomized trial or well-designed observational studies. Level C recommendations reflect expert consensus, clinical experience, or case series. Off-label recommendations always include the evidence level so you can make informed prescribing decisions in partnership with your patients.

Where clinical guidelines from major organizations (APA, VA/DoD, NICE, CANMAT, WFSBP) diverge on a recommendation, this book presents both positions and identifies the more conservative versus more aggressive approach. You will never be told that a single answer exists when legitimate clinical disagreement persists.

Part I: Foundations for Psychiatric Prescribing

Chapters 1 through 4: Neuroscience, Pharmacokinetics, Pharmacogenomics, Assessment

Chapter 1.0: Neuroscience Prescribing Essentials

Every medication you prescribe alters neurotransmission. Every side effect your patient reports traces back to receptor activity in a specific brain region. Every dangerous drug combination you avoid reflects an understanding of how overlapping pharmacodynamic mechanisms produce toxicity. The neuroscience in this chapter is not academic background. It is the operating system that runs every prescribing decision you make.

This chapter provides the neurobiological foundation you need to select medications rationally, predict side effects before they occur, and understand why certain drug combinations are synergistic while others are lethal. You do not need to memorize every receptor subtype. You need to understand the clinical logic that connects brain circuitry to the prescriptions you write.

1.1 Neurotransmitter Systems Overview

The brain communicates through chemical messengers, and psychiatric medications work by modifying these communication systems. Five neurotransmitter systems dominate psychopharmacology: serotonin, dopamine, norepinephrine, GABA/glutamate, and acetylcholine. Two additional systems, histamine and orexin, play supporting roles that explain sedation profiles and emerging sleep pharmacology.

Serotonin is the most targeted neurotransmitter in psychiatric prescribing. Serotonergic neurons originate primarily in the raphe nuclei of the brainstem and project widely throughout the cortex, limbic system, hypothalamus, and spinal cord (Stahl, 2021). The clinical relevance lies not in serotonin as a single entity but in its receptor subtypes. The 5-HT1A receptor functions as both a presynaptic autoreceptor (regulating serotonin release) and a postsynaptic receptor in cortical and limbic regions. Stimulation of 5-HT1A receptors is associated with anxiolytic and antidepressant effects, which is precisely why buspirone (a 5-HT1A partial agonist) reduces anxiety and why SSRIs take weeks to work. The therapeutic delay with SSRIs occurs because presynaptic 5-HT1A autoreceptors must desensitize before serotonin transmission is fully enhanced (Blier, 2014).

The 5-HT2A receptor tells a different clinical story. Blockade of 5-HT2A receptors reduces psychotic symptoms (the mechanism underlying atypical antipsychotics), improves sleep architecture, and may enhance dopamine release in the prefrontal cortex (Meltzer, 1999). When you prescribe quetiapine at low doses for insomnia, 5-HT2A antagonism is doing the work. When you choose an atypical antipsychotic over a typical one because your patient cannot tolerate extrapyramidal symptoms, you are leveraging the 5-HT2A/D2 receptor ratio.

The 5-HT2C receptor influences appetite and weight. Blockade of 5-HT2C (seen with mirtazapine and olanzapine) produces weight gain. Stimulation of 5-HT2C (seen with lorcaserin, now withdrawn) reduces appetite. The 5-HT3 receptor, when activated, produces nausea, which is why SSRIs cause GI distress in the first weeks of treatment. And the 5-HT7 receptor, increasingly recognized for its role in circadian rhythm regulation, may explain some of the sleep-modulating effects of certain antidepressants (Celada et al., 2013).

Dopamine operates through four major pathways, and understanding each one predicts both therapeutic effects and side effects of every antipsychotic you prescribe. The **mesolimbic pathway** runs from the ventral tegmental area to the nucleus accumbens. Hyperactivity in this pathway is associated with positive psychotic symptoms: hallucinations, delusions, disorganized thought. All antipsychotics reduce mesolimbic dopamine transmission, and this is the therapeutic target (Howes & Kapur, 2009).

The **mesocortical pathway** projects from the VTA to the prefrontal cortex. Hypoactivity here is associated with negative symptoms of schizophrenia and cognitive deficits. Here lies the cruel paradox of antipsychotic prescribing: blocking D2 receptors in the mesolimbic pathway helps positive symptoms, but blocking D2 in the mesocortical pathway can worsen negative symptoms and cognitive function (Stahl, 2021). Atypical antipsychotics partially solve this problem through their serotonin-dopamine activity ratio.

The **nigrostriatal pathway** connects the substantia nigra to the dorsal striatum and controls motor function. Block D2 receptors here and you produce extrapyramidal symptoms: dystonia, akathisia, parkinsonism, and with chronic exposure, tardive dyskinesia. The **tuberoinfundibular pathway** connects the hypothalamus to the pituitary. D2 blockade in this pathway removes the inhibition on prolactin release, producing hyperprolactinemia, galactorrhea, and menstrual irregularities (Sadock et al., 2015).

Norepinephrine originates in the locus coeruleus and projects to the prefrontal cortex, limbic system, and cerebellum. This system modulates attention, arousal, mood, and the stress response. SNRIs like venlafaxine and duloxetine enhance norepinephrine transmission alongside serotonin. The norepinephrine component is clinically relevant for patients presenting with fatigue-predominant depression, concentration difficulties, or comorbid chronic pain (Nutt, 2008). Atomoxetine, a selective norepinephrine reuptake inhibitor, treats ADHD through this same system without stimulant-class risks.

GABA and glutamate represent the brain's primary inhibitory and excitatory systems, respectively. GABA-A receptor potentiation is the mechanism of benzodiazepines and Z-drugs. Glutamate modulation is the mechanism behind ketamine, esketamine, and memantine. The emerging understanding of glutamate's role in mood disorders has produced some of the most significant pharmacological advances in recent years, including the NMDA receptor antagonist dextromethorphan/bupropion (Auvelity) for depression (Sanacora et al., 2012).

Acetylcholine operates through muscarinic and nicotinic receptor subtypes. Muscarinic blockade produces the anticholinergic side effects clinicians encounter daily: dry mouth, constipation, urinary retention, blurred vision, cognitive impairment. The anticholinergic burden of a medication regimen becomes especially important in geriatric prescribing. And muscarinic agonism is the novel mechanism behind Cobenfy (xanomeline/trospium), the first non-dopaminergic antipsychotic approved in decades (Stahl, 2021).

Histamine H1 receptor blockade produces sedation and weight gain. This explains the sedating profiles of quetiapine, olanzapine, and mirtazapine. **Orexin** is a hypothalamic neuropeptide that promotes wakefulness. Dual orexin receptor antagonists (suvorexant, lemborexant) represent a newer pharmacological approach to insomnia that avoids GABA-A receptor modulation entirely (Herring et al., 2012).

1.2 Receptor Pharmacology Applied

Understanding receptor pharmacology at the prescribing level means knowing four categories of drug-receptor interaction: full agonists, antagonists, partial agonists, and inverse agonists.

A **full agonist** binds a receptor and produces maximum response. Morphine at the mu-opioid receptor is a classic example. In psychiatric prescribing, buspirone acts as a full agonist at presynaptic 5-HT1A receptors. A **full antagonist** binds the receptor and blocks it, producing no intrinsic activity while preventing endogenous neurotransmitters from binding. Haloperidol at the D2 receptor is the prototypical example: it blocks dopamine completely, which produces robust antipsychotic effects alongside significant extrapyramidal side effects (Stahl, 2021).

A **partial agonist** is where prescribing becomes more nuanced. Partial agonists bind the receptor and produce a submaximal response. In environments of high neurotransmitter activity, they function as functional antagonists (reducing excessive stimulation). In environments of low activity, they function as functional agonists (providing baseline stimulation). Aripiprazole is the clearest clinical example. As a D2 partial agonist, it reduces dopamine transmission where it is excessive (mesolimbic pathway, reducing psychosis) while maintaining some dopamine activity where it is deficient (mesocortical pathway, potentially sparing cognition). This is also why aripiprazole causes less prolactin elevation and fewer EPS compared to full D2 antagonists (Shapiro et al., 2003).

Allosteric modulation adds another layer. Benzodiazepines do not directly activate the GABA-A receptor. They bind at an allosteric site and enhance the receptor's response to GABA that is already present. This is why benzodiazepines have a ceiling effect on sedation (unlike barbiturates, which can directly open the chloride channel) and why they require endogenous GABA to function.

The **therapeutic window** concept ties receptor pharmacology to clinical dosing. Some medications are more effective at moderate receptor occupancy than at full occupancy. D2 receptor occupancy between 60% and 80% is associated with antipsychotic efficacy. Below 60%, therapeutic effects are minimal. Above 80%, extrapyramidal side effects emerge sharply (Kapur et al., 2000). This principle guides dosing: enough to occupy the therapeutic range, not so much that side effect thresholds are crossed.

Consider the case of Marcus (composite example), a 34-year-old male presenting with first-episode psychosis. He reports auditory hallucinations, paranoid ideation, and social withdrawal over six months. His BMI is 32 and his fasting glucose is 112 mg/dL. Choosing an antipsychotic requires matching receptor pharmacology to this patient's clinical profile. Olanzapine would be highly effective for psychotic symptoms but carries substantial metabolic risk given his baseline. Aripiprazole, as a D2 partial agonist with minimal H1 and 5-HT2C activity, offers antipsychotic efficacy with a far more favorable metabolic profile. The receptor pharmacology drives the clinical decision. His metabolic risk factors steer you toward a weight-neutral agent, and understanding which receptors produce which side effects makes the choice rational rather than reflexive.

1.3 Mechanism to Medication Selection

The translation from neuroscience to prescribing becomes concrete when you can connect a patient's symptom cluster to the neurotransmitter system most likely involved, then select a medication that targets that system.

Consider a patient presenting with depression characterized by persistent sadness, anhedonia, insomnia, poor concentration, and fatigue. An SSRI targets serotonin broadly and is appropriate as first-line treatment. But if the dominant symptoms are fatigue, psychomotor retardation, and difficulty concentrating (with less prominent sadness and anxiety), the noradrenergic and dopaminergic components of the clinical picture suggest that an SNRI or bupropion might address the symptom cluster more precisely (Nutt, 2008). This is not guesswork. It is the clinical application of neurotransmitter pharmacology.

Now consider why mechanism knowledge prevents dangerous combinations. A patient on sertraline (an SSRI) who is prescribed tramadol for pain faces serotonin syndrome risk because both medications increase serotonergic transmission through different mechanisms. One blocks reuptake; the other has direct serotonergic activity. The overlap is pharmacodynamic, not pharmacokinetic, and understanding this distinction changes prescribing behavior (Boyer & Shannon, 2005).

Consider the case of Elena (identifying details changed for confidentiality), a 42-year-old woman presenting with major depression, chronic lower back pain, and significant fatigue. She has failed a 12-week trial of sertraline 200mg, which improved her mood modestly but did nothing for her pain or energy level. Her fatigue is so severe that she describes herself as "moving through mud" by early afternoon. She reports no anxiety symptoms.

Her symptom profile points toward serotonergic, noradrenergic, and potentially dopaminergic deficiency. Sertraline addressed the serotonergic component but missed the others. Switching to duloxetine (an SNRI with FDA approval for both MDD and chronic pain conditions) targets serotonin and norepinephrine simultaneously, addressing her mood, pain, and potentially her fatigue through noradrenergic activation. If fatigue persists, augmentation with bupropion adds dopaminergic and additional noradrenergic activity. The decision tree follows the neurobiology.

This is the clinical logic that runs throughout this book. You do not need to recall every receptor affinity table. You need the framework: identify the dominant symptom cluster, connect it to the neurotransmitter system most likely involved, select a medication that targets that system, and then monitor for both therapeutic response and predictable side effects based on the medication's receptor profile.

1.4 Clinical Implications

The neuroscience foundation covered in this chapter is not theoretical background you can afford to forget. Every chapter that follows builds on these principles. When you reach the decision tree for treatment-resistant depression in section 5.4, the augmentation strategies will make sense because you understand how aripiprazole's D2 partial agonism complements an SSRI's serotonin reuptake inhibition. When you evaluate a patient's akathisia on risperidone, you will connect that symptom to nigrostriatal D2 blockade and know that dose reduction or switching to a lower-EPS-risk agent is the appropriate response.

As you move forward into Chapter 2.0, where we examine how the body processes these medications (absorption, metabolism, elimination), keep in mind that the pharmacodynamics covered here determine *what* a drug does, while the pharmacokinetics we are about to explore determine *how much* drug is available to do it. Both sides are necessary for safe, effective prescribing.

1.5 Key Takeaways

Psychiatric medications work by modifying neurotransmitter systems. The five primary systems (serotonin, dopamine, norepinephrine, GABA/glutamate, and acetylcholine) each produce distinct clinical effects and side effect profiles when pharmacologically targeted. Serotonin receptor subtypes explain why SSRIs cause nausea (5-HT3), sexual dysfunction (descending spinal serotonergic pathways), and weight changes (5-HT2C). Dopamine's four pathways predict why antipsychotics treat psychosis (mesolimbic blockade) but produce movement disorders (nigrostriatal blockade) and prolactin elevation (tuberoinfundibular blockade). Partial agonism at D2 receptors offers a more nuanced pharmacological approach with potentially fewer side effects than full antagonism. Allosteric modulation at GABA-A explains benzodiazepine pharmacology and its ceiling effect. Connecting symptom clusters to neurotransmitter systems allows rational medication selection based on mechanism, not trial and error.

Chapter 2.0: Pharmacokinetic Clinical Principles

You can select the perfect medication based on receptor pharmacology, but if you don't understand how the body absorbs, distributes, metabolizes, and eliminates that medication, your prescribing will be unpredictable. A 50-year-old patient on fluoxetine who starts omeprazole may experience an unexpected change in drug levels. A patient who smokes a pack a day and takes olanzapine will need a dose adjustment if they quit. A switch from one SSRI to another requires a washout period that depends entirely on half-life. Pharmacokinetics is the clinical math behind every dose, every interaction, and every transition in psychiatric prescribing.

2.1 ADME in Psychiatric Practice

Absorption is the process by which a medication enters the bloodstream. Most psychiatric medications are administered orally and absorbed through the gastrointestinal tract. Clinically, this matters in several ways. Lurasidone must be taken with at least 350 calories of food to achieve adequate absorption; without food, bioavailability drops by approximately 50%, rendering the prescribed dose sub-therapeutic (Stahl, 2021). Ziprasidone has a similar food requirement. Long-acting injectable antipsychotics bypass absorption variability entirely, which is one reason they improve adherence outcomes (Correll et al., 2016).

Distribution describes how a medication spreads through body compartments. Lipophilicity determines if a drug crosses the blood-brain barrier effectively and and if it accumulates in adipose tissue. Highly lipophilic medications like diazepam distribute into fat stores and have prolonged clinical effects in obese patients. Volume of distribution affects dosing calculations for medications like lithium, where narrow therapeutic windows make precise dosing essential (Malhi et al., 2017).

Metabolism is where the prescriber's daily clinical decisions concentrate. The liver's cytochrome P450 enzyme system is responsible for Phase I metabolism of the majority of psychiatric medications. We will address this in detail in section 2.2. Metabolism determines a drug's effective half-life, the duration of its clinical effects, and the potential for drug-drug interactions.

Elimination occurs primarily through renal excretion. Lithium is the most clinically significant example because it is eliminated entirely by the kidneys without hepatic metabolism. Any change in renal function (dehydration, NSAIDs, ACE inhibitors, thiazide diuretics) directly affects lithium levels and can precipitate toxicity (Malhi et al., 2017). Gabapentin and pregabalin are also renally eliminated, requiring dose adjustment in renal impairment.

Half-life is the pharmacokinetic parameter most directly relevant to daily prescribing. It takes approximately 4 to 5 half-lives for a medication to reach steady state, and the same duration for a medication to wash out after discontinuation. Fluoxetine's active metabolite norfluoxetine has a half-life of 4 to 16 days, which is why fluoxetine requires a 5-week washout before starting an MAOI (Hiemke & Hartter, 2000). Sertraline's half-life of approximately 26 hours means steady state is reached in about 5 to 7 days, and washout is achieved in roughly a week. This practical knowledge guides every cross-taper and switching protocol.

Consider the case of Priya (composite example), a 38-year-old woman who has been stable on paroxetine 40mg for three years and now wants to switch to a medication with fewer sexual side effects. She and her provider agree to trial bupropion. The switching strategy must account for paroxetine's pharmacokinetics. Paroxetine has a half-life of approximately 21 hours but is notorious for discontinuation syndrome because of its potent serotonin reuptake inhibition and lack of active metabolites. A direct switch would leave her without serotonergic coverage for days before bupropion (which has no serotonergic activity) reaches steady state. The clinical plan: cross-taper over two weeks, reducing paroxetine by 25% per week while titrating bupropion upward. The pharmacokinetic rationale drives the transition timeline.

2.2 CYP450 Prescribing Reference

The cytochrome P450 system is a family of liver enzymes that metabolize the majority of psychiatric medications. Four enzymes handle the bulk of the work: CYP2D6, CYP2C19, CYP3A4, and CYP1A2. A fifth, CYP2B6, metabolizes bupropion specifically (Preskorn, 2013).

CYP2D6 metabolizes numerous antidepressants (fluoxetine, paroxetine, venlafaxine, nortriptyline), antipsychotics (risperidone, aripiprazole, haloperidol, thioridazine), and atomoxetine. This enzyme shows significant genetic polymorphism, which is covered in Chapter 3.0. Clinically, fluoxetine and paroxetine are potent CYP2D6 inhibitors. Adding either to a regimen that includes a CYP2D6 substrate (such as aripiprazole) will increase the substrate's blood levels, potentially producing side effects at otherwise therapeutic doses (Stahl, 2021).

CYP2C19 metabolizes citalopram, escitalopram, sertraline (partially), diazepam, and certain proton pump inhibitors. Genetic variation in CYP2C19 is clinically meaningful: poor metabolizers accumulate higher levels of citalopram and escitalopram, which increases QTc prolongation risk. The FDA has recommended dose ceilings for citalopram that reflect this pharmacogenomic reality (Hicks et al., 2015).

CYP3A4 metabolizes quetiapine, lurasidone, buspirone, alprazolam, and midazolam. This enzyme is inhibited by ketoconazole, erythromycin, grapefruit juice, and certain HIV protease inhibitors. It is induced by carbamazepine, phenytoin, and St. John's Wort. A patient on quetiapine who starts carbamazepine will see quetiapine levels drop significantly due to CYP3A4 induction, potentially losing antipsychotic coverage (Preskorn, 2013).

CYP1A2 metabolizes clozapine, olanzapine, and duloxetine. Smoking (specifically the polycyclic aromatic hydrocarbons in cigarette smoke, not nicotine itself) is a potent CYP1A2 inducer. A patient on clozapine who quits smoking will experience rising clozapine levels over days to weeks, potentially reaching toxic concentrations. Fluvoxamine is a potent CYP1A2 inhibitor and should generally be avoided with clozapine (Stahl, 2021).

2.3 Critical Drug Interactions

Some drug interactions in psychiatric prescribing carry life-threatening consequences. The prescriber who understands these interactions prevents emergencies.

Serotonin syndrome results from excessive serotonergic activity and presents as a triad of autonomic instability (hyperthermia, tachycardia, diaphoresis), neuromuscular hyperactivity (clonus, hyperreflexia, tremor), and altered mental status. High-risk combinations include any SSRI or SNRI with an MAOI, tramadol, linezolid, methylene blue, or certain triptans. The Hunter Criteria provide the most sensitive and specific diagnostic framework (Boyer & Shannon, 2005). Prevention is straightforward: maintain a minimum 14-day washout between MAOIs and serotonergic agents (5 weeks for fluoxetine due to norfluoxetine's prolonged half-life).

QTc prolongation is a pharmacodynamic interaction that can produce torsades de pointes and sudden cardiac death. High-risk psychotropics include ziprasidone, thioridazine, IV haloperidol, and high-dose citalopram. Combining QTc-prolonging agents increases risk synergistically. Baseline ECG is indicated before starting high-risk agents, and serial monitoring is warranted when combinations are unavoidable (Beach et al., 2013).

Lithium toxicity is precipitated by pharmacokinetic interactions that reduce lithium clearance. NSAIDs, ACE inhibitors, and thiazide diuretics all decrease lithium elimination. Dehydration from any cause (illness, heat, inadequate fluid intake) concentrates lithium levels. Patients on lithium need to understand these interactions, and prescribers need to check lithium levels whenever a new interacting medication is added or renal function changes (Malhi et al., 2017).

The **valproate-lamotrigine interaction** is pharmacokinetic: valproate inhibits the glucuronidation of lamotrigine, increasing lamotrigine levels and the risk of Stevens-Johnson syndrome. When co-prescribing, lamotrigine titration must be halved (standard titration: 25mg daily for 2 weeks; with valproate: 25mg every other day for 2 weeks). This interaction is especially relevant in bipolar maintenance, where both medications are commonly used (Stahl, 2021).

Carbamazepine is a potent pan-inducer of CYP3A4, CYP2C9, CYP1A2, and UGT enzymes. It accelerates the metabolism of oral contraceptives (risking unplanned pregnancy), many antipsychotics, benzodiazepines, and lamotrigine. Adding carbamazepine to an existing regimen is one of the most interaction-dense changes a prescriber can make, and it demands a systematic review of every co-prescribed medication (Preskorn, 2013).

Consider the case of Diego (identifying details changed), a 56-year-old man with bipolar I disorder stabilized on lithium 900mg and quetiapine 400mg. He develops a seizure disorder and his neurologist prescribes carbamazepine. The prescribing implications cascade immediately. Carbamazepine induces CYP3A4, which will lower quetiapine levels substantially. It also increases renal lithium clearance in some patients and has its own mood-stabilizing properties that overlap pharmacodynamically with lithium. The prescriber must anticipate quetiapine dose adjustment upward, closer monitoring of lithium levels, and potential for additive CNS effects. A single new medication produces three distinct interaction concerns. This is why CYP450 literacy is not optional.

2.4 Synthesis and Clinical Application

Pharmacokinetics translates directly into prescribing safety. Every dose titration, every medication switch, every addition of a new drug to an existing regimen should prompt two questions. First: does this new medication share metabolic pathways with anything my patient is already taking? Second: does this change alter the absorption, distribution, metabolism, or elimination of existing medications?

The CYP450 tables in Chapter 24.0 are designed for rapid reference during clinical encounters. When you are sitting with a patient and considering a medication change, those tables answer the interaction question in under 30 seconds. As we move into Chapter 3.0 on pharmacogenomics, you will see how genetic variation in these same CYP450 enzymes produces the wide inter-individual variability in medication response that you observe every day in clinical practice.

Chapter 3.0: Pharmacogenomics in Practice

Your patient has failed three adequate antidepressant trials. Each time, you selected a reasonable medication at an appropriate dose for an adequate duration, and each time, the result was the same: minimal improvement or intolerable side effects. Before concluding that this is true treatment resistance, consider the possibility that your patient metabolizes one or more of those medications in a way that standard dosing does not accommodate. Pharmacogenomic testing can reveal this pattern, and it is increasingly accessible, increasingly covered by insurance, and increasingly relevant to everyday prescribing.

3.1 Ordering and Indications

Pharmacogenomic (PGx) testing analyzes variations in genes that encode drug-metabolizing enzymes, primarily the CYP450 family discussed in section 2.2. The clinical question is straightforward: does this patient metabolize psychiatric medications at a rate that standard dosing assumes?

Testing is most clinically useful in specific scenarios. Patients who have failed two or more adequate medication trials warrant testing to rule out pharmacokinetic explanations for nonresponse (Bousman et al., 2021). Patients who experience severe or unexpected side effects at standard doses may be poor metabolizers who accumulate drug levels beyond the therapeutic window. Patients on complex polypharmacy regimens benefit from testing because genetic predictions interact with drug-drug inhibition effects (a concept called phenoconversion, which we will address in section 3.2). Patients beginning medications with narrow therapeutic indices, such as tricyclic antidepressants or clozapine, may benefit from preemptive testing.

Available commercial panels (GeneSight, Genomind, Tempus, OneOme) typically test CYP2D6, CYP2C19, CYP2C9, CYP2B6, CYP3A4, and pharmacodynamic genes such as SLC6A4 (serotonin transporter) and HTR2A (serotonin 2A receptor). The pharmacokinetic results (CYP enzyme status) have the strongest evidence base and the most actionable clinical guidelines. The pharmacodynamic results remain less robustly supported in clinical trials, though research is advancing (Zeier et al., 2018).

Insurance coverage has expanded significantly. Medicare covers PGx testing under the MolDX (Molecular Diagnostic Services) program when medical necessity criteria are met, typically requiring documentation of prior treatment failure or adverse drug reactions. Most major commercial insurers now cover testing in similar clinical circumstances. Out-of-pocket costs for patients without coverage typically range from $250 to $500, and many testing companies offer financial assistance programs (Bousman et al., 2021).

3.2 Interpreting Test Results

Test results classify patients by metabolizer phenotype for each enzyme tested. The four standard categories for CYP2D6 and CYP2C19 are: **poor metabolizer** (PM, little to no enzyme activity), **intermediate metabolizer** (IM, reduced activity), **normal metabolizer** (NM, previously called extensive metabolizer, with typical activity), and **ultra-rapid metabolizer** (UM, increased activity). Each phenotype has direct prescribing implications.

A CYP2D6 poor metabolizer will accumulate higher-than-expected blood levels of medications metabolized by 2D6 at standard doses. For aripiprazole, CPIC guidelines recommend reducing the starting dose by approximately 50% in CYP2D6 PMs (Hicks et al., 2015). For codeine (a prodrug requiring CYP2D6 conversion to morphine), poor metabolizers get no analgesic effect because the active metabolite is never formed. Conversely, CYP2D6 ultra-rapid metabolizers convert codeine too rapidly, producing dangerously high morphine levels.

For CYP2C19, poor metabolizers accumulate higher levels of citalopram and escitalopram. CPIC guidelines recommend a 50% dose reduction for citalopram in CYP2C19 PMs, capping the dose at 20mg daily to avoid QTc prolongation. Sertraline, which uses multiple metabolic pathways, is less affected but still warrants monitoring (Hicks et al., 2015).

HLA screening is a separate but related pharmacogenomic consideration. HLA-B*1502 testing is recommended before prescribing carbamazepine or oxcarbazepine to patients of Southeast Asian descent due to elevated risk of Stevens-Johnson syndrome and toxic epidermal necrolysis. HLA-A*3101 testing extends this screening to broader populations with carbamazepine use (Leckband et al., 2013). These are binary tests: the allele is present or absent, and a positive result is generally a contraindication to prescribing the associated medication.

Phenoconversion is a concept that connects pharmacogenomics to the drug interaction principles from Chapter 2.0. A patient may have a normal CYP2D6 genotype, but if they are concurrently taking fluoxetine (a potent CYP2D6 inhibitor), their functional phenotype shifts to poor metabolizer status. Their genetic test says "normal metabolizer," but their actual drug-metabolizing capacity is impaired by the interacting medication. This is why PGx results cannot be interpreted in isolation. They must be contextualized within the patient's current medication list and clinical circumstances (Mostafa et al., 2022).

Consider the case of Aisha (composite example), a 29-year-old woman with major depression who has failed adequate trials of sertraline (200mg for 10 weeks), escitalopram (20mg for 8 weeks), and venlafaxine XR (225mg for 10 weeks). Side effects were minimal with each trial, but therapeutic response was negligible. PGx testing reveals she is a CYP2C19 ultra-rapid metabolizer. This finding explains the pattern: she was metabolizing the SSRIs too quickly, never achieving adequate plasma levels at standard doses. The clinical adjustment: select a medication less dependent on CYP2C19 metabolism (such as duloxetine, primarily metabolized by CYP1A2 and CYP2D6), or consider a higher-than-standard dose of a CYP2C19 substrate with close monitoring. Her "treatment resistance" was pharmacokinetic, not pharmacodynamic.

3.3 Clinical Application

Applying PGx results to prescribing decisions follows the guidelines published by CPIC and the Dutch Pharmacogenetics Working Group (DPWG). As of 2024, CPIC and DPWG have collectively published dosing guidelines for 14 antidepressants, seven antipsychotics, three anticonvulsant/mood stabilizers, and atomoxetine for ADHD (Brown et al., 2019; Hicks et al., 2015).

The practical application follows a three-step process. First, identify the patient's metabolizer status for the relevant enzyme. Second, determine if the medication you are considering is a substrate of that enzyme. Third, consult the CPIC guideline for specific dose modifications or alternative medication recommendations.

For example, a patient who is a CYP2D6 poor metabolizer being started on nortriptyline would receive a 50% dose reduction per CPIC guidelines, with therapeutic drug monitoring to guide further titration. A CYP2D6 ultra-rapid metabolizer being started on the same medication might need an alternative agent entirely, because achieving therapeutic levels may require supraphysiological doses (Hicks et al., 2017).

It is equally important to understand what PGx testing cannot tell you. It does not predict which medication will work best for a specific diagnosis. It does not account for pharmacodynamic variability (receptor sensitivity, signal transduction efficiency). And it does not replace clinical judgment. A normal metabolizer can still fail to respond to a well-chosen medication for reasons unrelated to metabolism (incorrect diagnosis, psychosocial factors, nonadherence). PGx testing narrows one variable. It does not solve the clinical puzzle by itself (Zeier et al., 2018).

Consider the case of James (identifying details changed), a 63-year-old man with bipolar I disorder requiring carbamazepine for mood stabilization after lamotrigine produced an allergic rash. Before prescribing carbamazepine, his provider orders HLA-B*1502 and HLA-A*3101 testing. His ancestry is Northern European. Testing returns negative for both alleles, and carbamazepine is initiated with standard titration and monitoring. Had either allele been positive, the provider would have selected an alternative mood stabilizer (valproate, lithium, or an atypical antipsychotic), and the test result would have prevented a potentially fatal dermatologic reaction.

3.4 Limitations and Future Directions

The evidence base for PGx-guided prescribing is stronger for pharmacokinetic genes (CYP enzymes) than for pharmacodynamic genes (receptor variants, transporter polymorphisms). The GUIDED trial, the largest randomized study of combinatorial PGx testing in depression, did not find statistically significant differences in response rates on its primary outcome measure, though secondary analyses showed improvement in certain subgroups (Greden et al., 2019). The PRIME Care trial in the VA system showed more promising results for medication selection guided by PGx data (Oslin et al., 2022).

Clinical decision support tools are evolving to integrate PGx results with drug interaction data at the point of care, addressing the phenoconversion problem and making results more actionable for busy prescribers. As the evidence base matures and costs continue to decline, preemptive PGx testing (testing before the first medication is prescribed, rather than after failures accumulate) may become standard practice.

3.5 Chapter Summary

Pharmacogenomic testing provides actionable information about how individual patients metabolize psychiatric medications. Testing is most useful after multiple treatment failures, severe unexplained side effects, or before initiating narrow-therapeutic-index medications. Results classify patients by metabolizer phenotype for key CYP450 enzymes, with CPIC and DPWG guidelines providing specific dose adjustments and alternative medication recommendations. HLA testing prevents life-threatening dermatologic reactions with carbamazepine and related agents. Phenoconversion (the discrepancy between genotype and functional phenotype caused by drug interactions) must be considered when interpreting results. PGx testing narrows pharmacokinetic variability but does not replace clinical judgment, accurate diagnosis, or attention to psychosocial factors.

Chapter 4.0: Medication Management Assessment

The 15-minute medication management visit is the clinical reality for most psychiatric prescribers. You do not have the luxury of a 50-minute intake at every follow-up. What you do have is a structured assessment framework that captures the essential clinical data needed to make safe prescribing decisions, monitor treatment response, screen for emergent risks, and document your reasoning. This chapter provides that framework.

4.1 Structured Rapid Assessment

A structured approach to the medication visit prevents the two most common errors: missing critical information because you relied on an unstructured conversation, and spending disproportionate time on history-taking while leaving no time for clinical decision-making.

The rapid mental status examination (MSE) for medication visits focuses on the elements most relevant to pharmacological management. Appearance and behavior: has the patient gained or lost visible weight? Are there signs of EPS, akathisia, or sedation? Mood and affect: does the patient's reported mood align with observed affect, and has it changed since last visit? Thought process and content: any psychotic symptoms, suicidal ideation, or concerning cognitive changes? These observations take less than two minutes when performed systematically and provide critical data that the patient may not spontaneously report (Sadock et al., 2015).

Standardized rating scales convert subjective reports into quantifiable data that track treatment response over time. The **PHQ-9** (Patient Health Questionnaire-9) measures depression severity on a 0 to 27 scale. A score reduction of 50% or greater indicates clinical response. A score of 5 or below indicates remission. Administering the PHQ-9 at every medication visit takes under three minutes and provides objective data for prescribing decisions (Kroenke et al., 2001).

The **GAD-7** (Generalized Anxiety Disorder-7) measures anxiety severity on a 0 to 21 scale with corresponding severity thresholds: 5-9 mild, 10-14 moderate, 15-21 severe. Like the PHQ-9, it is brief, validated, and directly useful for tracking response to anxiolytic medication (Spitzer et al., 2006).

The **MDQ** (Mood Disorder Questionnaire) screens for bipolar spectrum disorders and should be administered when there is any clinical suspicion of bipolarity in a patient presenting with depression. A positive screen does not confirm diagnosis but prompts further assessment before prescribing an antidepressant without mood stabilizer coverage (Hirschfeld et al., 2000).

The **PCL-5** (PTSD Checklist for DSM-5) is a 20-item self-report measure tracking PTSD symptom severity. It is especially useful for monitoring response to prazosin for nightmares and SSRI/SNRI treatment for daytime PTSD symptoms (Bovin et al., 2016).

The **Columbia Suicide Severity Rating Scale (C-SSRS)** provides structured suicide risk assessment that is more clinically reliable than unstructured inquiry. It distinguishes between passive ideation, active ideation without plan, active ideation with plan, and preparatory behavior. Integration of the C-SSRS into every medication visit creates a documented risk assessment that supports clinical decision-making and liability protection (Posner et al., 2011).

Consider the case of Nicole (composite example), a 27-year-old woman presenting for a 4-week follow-up after starting sertraline 50mg for moderate major depression. Her PHQ-9 at baseline was 17 (moderately severe). Today her PHQ-9 is 14, a 17.6% reduction, which falls below the 50% response threshold. However, she reports improved sleep and appetite, and her affect is brighter than at her last visit. She denies suicidal ideation on the C-SSRS. The rating scale data and clinical observation together inform the decision: optimize the dose to 100mg rather than switch or augment, because partial early improvement at a sub-therapeutic dose suggests the mechanism is correct and the dose is insufficient. Without the PHQ-9 anchoring the conversation, this visit might have concluded with either premature satisfaction ("I feel a little better") or premature switching.

4.2 Monitoring Protocols

Baseline and ongoing laboratory monitoring varies by medication class and is one of the most frequently under-performed aspects of psychiatric prescribing. Every medication initiation should prompt the question: what do I need to measure before starting, and what do I need to track over time?

Metabolic monitoring is required for all patients starting atypical antipsychotics. The APA/ADA consensus guidelines recommend baseline measurements of weight, BMI, waist circumference, fasting glucose, fasting lipid panel, and blood pressure. Weight should be reassessed at 4 weeks, 8 weeks, 12 weeks, and quarterly thereafter. Fasting glucose and lipid panel should be rechecked at 12 weeks and annually. Patients on olanzapine and clozapine require the most vigilant metabolic monitoring due to their highest-risk profiles (American Diabetes Association et al., 2004).

Cardiac monitoring with baseline ECG is indicated before starting medications with known QTc prolongation risk: ziprasidone, thioridazine, IV haloperidol, citalopram (especially at doses above 40mg or in patients over 60), and escitalopram (at higher doses). A QTc above 500 milliseconds or an increase of more than 60 milliseconds from baseline warrants immediate medication reassessment (Beach et al., 2013).

Lithium monitoring requires baseline renal function (BUN, creatinine), thyroid function (TSH), calcium, and ECG. Lithium levels should be checked 5 to 7 days after initiation or dose change (allowing steady state to be reached), with a target trough level of 0.6 to 1.2 mEq/L for acute treatment and 0.6 to 0.8 mEq/L for maintenance. Renal and thyroid function should be monitored every 6 months during stable maintenance (Malhi et al., 2017).

Valproate monitoring includes baseline hepatic function (LFTs), CBC with platelets, and for women of reproductive age, a pregnancy test. Therapeutic levels range from 50 to 125 mcg/mL. LFTs should be checked at baseline, monthly for the first 6 months, and periodically thereafter. Ammonia levels should be checked if the patient develops unexplained lethargy or confusion (Stahl, 2021).

Clozapine monitoring has been simplified with the 2025 elimination of the Clozapine REMS program. However, the risk of severe neutropenia remains, and ANC monitoring continues to be clinically required. Baseline ANC must be at least 1500/mcL (1000/mcL for patients with benign ethnic neutropenia). Weekly ANC monitoring continues for the first 6 months, biweekly for months 6 through 12, and monthly thereafter for the duration of treatment (Stahl, 2021).

4.3 Risk Assessment Integration

Risk assessment is not a separate activity performed at the end of the visit. It is woven throughout the medication management encounter. Three domains require systematic screening at every visit: suicide risk, substance use, and reproductive risk.

Suicide risk assessment is especially pertinent during medication changes, because both improvement (restored energy enabling action on existing ideation) and worsening (medication failure or side effects) can shift risk. The C-SSRS provides structured assessment. The FDA black box warning on antidepressants for patients under 25 requires explicit documentation of suicidal ideation monitoring during the first weeks of treatment. Lithium's anti-suicidal properties make it a consideration in patients with mood disorders and elevated baseline suicide risk (Cipriani et al., 2013).

Substance use screening using the AUDIT-C (for alcohol) should be routine. Active substance use affects medication selection (avoid benzodiazepines in patients with substance use disorders), medication metabolism (smoking induces CYP1A2; alcohol affects hepatic function), and treatment response (active use undermines most pharmacological interventions). A brief screen takes under one minute and may fundamentally change the prescribing plan.

Pregnancy risk assessment must occur at every visit for patients of reproductive age who are taking teratogenic medications. Valproate carries the highest teratogenic risk among commonly prescribed psychiatric medications, with neural tube defect rates of 1 to 2% and neurodevelopmental effects in up to 30 to 40% of exposed pregnancies (Tomson et al., 2018). Lithium carries cardiac teratogenicity risk (Ebstein's anomaly, though the absolute risk is lower than historically reported). Carbamazepine is a known teratogen. Contraception status should be documented, and preconception counseling should be offered proactively.

Consider the case of Sofia (identifying details changed), a 31-year-old woman with bipolar II disorder maintained on valproate 1000mg and quetiapine 200mg. She presents at a routine medication visit and mentions she is considering starting a family within the next year. This information immediately triggers a prescribing reassessment. Valproate's teratogenicity makes it incompatible with planned pregnancy. The prescriber initiates a transition plan: cross-taper valproate to lamotrigine (the preferred mood stabilizer in pregnancy) over 6 to 8 weeks while ensuring mood stability at each step. Folic acid supplementation at 4mg daily is started immediately. She is counseled to continue effective contraception until the transition is complete and stable for at least one full mood cycle. Without systematic pregnancy risk screening at the medication visit, this conversation might not have happened until the pregnancy was already established, leaving far fewer safe options.

4.4 Integrating Assessment and Prescribing

The assessment framework in this chapter creates the foundation for every prescribing decision in the chapters that follow. When you reach the decision tree for treatment-resistant depression in section 5.4, the PHQ-9 scores from serial visits will define where your patient falls on the response continuum. When you manage a patient on clozapine, the monitoring protocol from section 4.2 will ensure you track ANC, metabolic parameters, and clinical signs systematically. When you are considering a medication change in a reproductive-age patient, the risk assessment framework from section 4.3 will prompt the contraception conversation before it becomes an emergency.

Part II of this book begins with Chapter 5.0, where the diagnosis-based prescribing framework takes over. Every algorithm and decision tree in Part II assumes that you have performed the assessment framework described here. The 15-minute visit is not much time. A structured approach ensures that every minute counts.

4.5 Essential Points

The 15-minute medication management visit requires structured assessment to capture critical clinical data efficiently. Standardized rating scales (PHQ-9, GAD-7, MDQ, PCL-5, C-SSRS) provide objective, trackable metrics that anchor prescribing decisions in quantifiable data rather than subjective impression alone. Baseline and ongoing laboratory monitoring is medication-class-specific and must be performed systematically: metabolic monitoring for antipsychotics, renal and thyroid monitoring for lithium, hepatic monitoring for valproate, and ANC monitoring for clozapine. Risk assessment for suicide, substance use, and pregnancy is not a separate activity but an integrated component of every medication visit. Documenting these assessments protects patients and supports clinical decision-making across the longitudinal course of treatment.

Part II: Diagnosis-Based Prescribing Guides

Chapters 5 through 17: The Clinical Core

Chapter 5.0: Major Depressive Disorder

A patient sits across from you and describes four months of persistent sadness, loss of interest in activities that once brought pleasure, disrupted sleep, difficulty concentrating at work, and a pervasive sense of worthlessness. The PHQ-9 score is 18. You have fifteen minutes to confirm the diagnosis, rule out critical differentials, and select a medication that matches this patient's specific clinical profile. This chapter gives you the decision architecture to do exactly that.

5.1 Diagnostic Confirmation

Before prescribing, confirm the diagnosis. DSM-5-TR requires five or more symptoms present during the same two-week period, with at least one being depressed mood or anhedonia. Symptoms must cause clinically significant distress or functional impairment and cannot be attributable to substance effects or another medical condition (American Psychiatric Association, 2022).

The prescribing-relevant specifiers matter. **Anxious distress** (present in over 50% of depressed outpatients) predicts slower treatment response and may warrant anxiolytic augmentation. **Mixed features** (concurrent subthreshold manic symptoms) signal bipolar risk and caution with antidepressant monotherapy. **Melancholic features** (profound anhedonia, psychomotor disturbance, early morning awakening, excessive guilt) may respond preferentially to SNRIs, TCAs, or ECT. **Atypical features** (mood reactivity, hypersomnia, leaden paralysis, rejection sensitivity) historically responded well to MAOIs, though SSRIs are now first-line. **Peripartum onset** triggers the prescribing considerations covered in Chapter 18.0. **Seasonal pattern** warrants light therapy integration (American Psychiatric Association, 2022).

The two critical rule-outs before prescribing an antidepressant are bipolar depression and medical causes. Administering the MDQ (discussed in section 4.1) screens for bipolar spectrum features. A positive screen should prompt further assessment before initiating antidepressant monotherapy, which risks triggering mania or rapid cycling in unrecognized bipolar disorder. Medical causes of depressive symptoms include hypothyroidism, anemia, vitamin B12 or folate deficiency, Cushing's syndrome, and medication effects (corticosteroids, interferon, beta-blockers). Baseline TSH and CBC are reasonable screening labs for new-onset depression (Sadock et al., 2015).

5.2 First-Line Medication Selection

SSRIs remain the first-line pharmacotherapy for major depressive disorder based on efficacy, tolerability, safety in overdose, and decades of clinical experience. The question is not if you should start an SSRI but which one, and the answer depends on the patient's symptom cluster, medical comorbidities, and side effect concerns.

Sertraline offers the broadest evidence base across depression subtypes and carries mild dopaminergic activity that may help with energy and motivation. It is generally weight-neutral and has favorable drug interaction profiles. Starting dose: 50mg daily, titrating to 100-200mg. **Escitalopram** is the most serotonin-selective SSRI with the cleanest pharmacology and fewest drug interactions, making it an excellent first choice in medically complex patients or those on multiple medications. Starting dose: 10mg daily, target 10-20mg. **Fluoxetine** has the longest half-life (including active metabolite norfluoxetine), making it forgiving of missed doses and producing the least discontinuation syndrome. However, it is a potent CYP2D6 inhibitor and activating, which may worsen insomnia or anxiety. Starting dose: 20mg daily (Cipriani et al., 2018).

Paroxetine is the most sedating SSRI and carries the highest rate of sexual dysfunction and weight gain. Its potent CYP2D6 inhibition and short half-life (producing significant discontinuation syndrome) make it a less favorable first choice for most patients. **Citalopram** has a dose-dependent QTc prolongation risk with a maximum recommended dose of 40mg (20mg in patients over 60 or with hepatic impairment). **Fluvoxamine** is primarily used for OCD rather than depression and is a potent CYP1A2 inhibitor, making it problematic with clozapine or olanzapine co-prescribing (Stahl, 2021).

When the dominant symptom profile includes significant fatigue, psychomotor retardation, or comorbid chronic pain, **SNRIs** may be more appropriate than SSRIs. **Duloxetine** (60-120mg) has FDA approval for MDD, GAD, diabetic neuropathy, fibromyalgia, and chronic musculoskeletal pain, making it efficient when these conditions co-occur. **Venlafaxine XR** (75-225mg) provides dose-dependent noradrenergic activity (primarily serotonergic below 150mg, adding norepinephrine above 150mg). Blood pressure monitoring is required, particularly above 225mg (Cipriani et al., 2018).

Bupropion (150-450mg) targets dopamine and norepinephrine with no serotonergic activity. It is the antidepressant of choice when sexual dysfunction must be avoided, and it is useful in fatigue-predominant depression, ADHD comorbidity, or smoking cessation. Seizure risk increases above 450mg daily and in patients with eating disorders or alcohol withdrawal. **Mirtazapine** (15-45mg) produces sedation and appetite stimulation through H1 and 5-HT2C antagonism, making it useful in underweight or insomnia-predominant patients. Paradoxically, sedation may decrease at higher doses as noradrenergic activity increases (Stahl, 2021).

Consider the case of Jamal (composite example), a 45-year-old man presenting with moderate MDD (PHQ-9: 16) characterized by persistent low mood, insomnia, poor appetite with 8-pound weight loss, and difficulty concentrating at work. He has no psychiatric history and takes lisinopril for hypertension. His symptom cluster of insomnia, appetite loss, and weight loss suggests mirtazapine could address multiple target symptoms simultaneously. Alternatively, sertraline offers the broadest evidence base with a favorable interaction profile alongside lisinopril. The decision tree proceeds: if sleep disturbance and weight loss are the most functionally impairing symptoms, mirtazapine is the targeted choice. If the prescriber prefers a more conservative first-line approach, sertraline with sleep hygiene counseling is appropriate. Either way, the medication selection is driven by the symptom profile, not by reflex.

5.3 Augmentation Strategies

When a patient achieves partial response (25-49% symptom reduction on PHQ-9) after an adequate trial (therapeutic dose for 6-8 weeks), augmentation is generally preferred over switching, because it preserves the partial benefit of the current medication.

Three atypical antipsychotics carry FDA approval for adjunctive treatment of MDD: **aripiprazole** (2-15mg), **brexpiprazole** (0.5-3mg), and **quetiapine XR** (150-300mg). Aripiprazole augmentation is the most extensively studied, with effect sizes of 0.3-0.4 compared to antidepressant monotherapy. Weight gain and akathisia are the primary limiting side effects. Brexpiprazole produces less akathisia than aripiprazole but similar weight gain. Quetiapine XR augmentation is effective but carries greater metabolic risk and sedation (Nelson & Papakostas, 2009).

Lumateperone (Caplyta) received FDA approval in 2025 as an adjunctive treatment for MDD in adults. It acts through serotonin, dopamine, and glutamate modulation with a favorable metabolic and movement disorder profile compared to other atypical antipsychotics used for augmentation. Dosing for MDD augmentation is 42mg daily (Durgam et al., 2024).

Lithium augmentation has robust evidence from multiple controlled trials and meta-analyses demonstrating response rates of

40-50% in antidepressant nonresponders. Despite strong evidence and anti-suicidal properties, lithium remains significantly underutilized for depression augmentation. Augmentation dosing targets levels of 0.4-0.8 mEq/L, lower than acute bipolar treatment levels (Nelson et al., 2014). **Thyroid hormone (T3) augmentation** at 25-50mcg daily has supporting evidence, particularly in women and patients with subclinical hypothyroidism. **Buspirone augmentation** adds 5-HT1A agonism and is weight-neutral, though evidence is more modest (Stahl, 2021).

5.4 Treatment Resistant Depression

Treatment-resistant depression (TRD) is defined as failure to respond adequately to two or more antidepressant trials of different classes at adequate doses for adequate duration (6-8 weeks each). Before concluding TRD, rule out **pseudo-resistance**: nonadherence, inadequate dosing, insufficient trial duration, unaddressed comorbidities (substance use, personality disorders, medical conditions), and pharmacokinetic factors (as discussed in section 3.2).

Esketamine (Spravato) received FDA approval as a monotherapy for TRD in 2025, expanding its prior indication that required concurrent oral antidepressant use. It is administered as a nasal spray under REMS-mandated observation in certified healthcare settings. Patients must be monitored for at least two hours after each dose due to dissociation, sedation, and blood pressure changes. The 84mg dose demonstrated effect sizes of 0.63 versus placebo in registration trials (Daly et al., 2019).

Auvelity (dextromethorphan/bupropion) targets NMDA glutamate receptors and sigma-1 receptors. It demonstrated faster onset of antidepressant effect compared to bupropion alone in clinical trials. Dosing starts at 45mg/105mg daily for three days, then increases to twice daily. It offers an oral TRD option that avoids the clinic-based administration required by esketamine (Iosifescu et al., 2022).

MAOIs remain underutilized options for TRD. Tranylcypromine and phenelzine require dietary tyramine restriction and carry drug interaction risks, but produce response rates of 50-70% in patients who have failed multiple other antidepressants. The transdermal selegiline patch (Emsam) at its lowest dose (6mg/24hr) bypasses first-pass gut MAO inhibition and does not require dietary restrictions, making it more practical (Stahl, 2021).

Consider the case of Rebecca (identifying details changed), a 52-year-old woman with recurrent MDD who has failed adequate trials of sertraline (200mg, 10 weeks), duloxetine (120mg, 8 weeks), and bupropion XL (450mg, 8 weeks). Aripiprazole augmentation of her most recent trial produced intolerable akathisia. Her PHQ-9 remains at 19. She has no cardiovascular contraindications and is motivated for treatment. The TRD decision tree branches: esketamine monotherapy (clinic-based, twice-weekly initially), Auvelity (oral, home-administered), or MAOI trial (dietary restrictions, washout period required from prior agents). Given her preference for home-administered treatment and reluctance to commit to twice-weekly clinic visits, Auvelity is initiated after appropriate washout from bupropion. The decision integrates patient preference with clinical evidence.

5.5 Monitoring and Maintenance

Response benchmarks guide prescribing decisions at defined intervals. At 2 weeks, look for at least 20% PHQ-9 improvement as an early signal of response. At 4 weeks, expect 25-50% improvement; if less than 25%, dose optimization is warranted. At 6-8 weeks, assess for full response (50% or greater reduction) or remission (PHQ-9 below 5). If response is inadequate after dose optimization, the decision tree moves to switching or augmentation (Rush et al., 2006).

Maintenance treatment duration depends on episode history. After a first episode, continue the effective antidepressant at the acute treatment dose for 6-12 months following remission. After two episodes, consider 2+ years of maintenance. After three or more episodes, indefinite maintenance is generally recommended (American Psychiatric Association, 2010).

Discontinuation syndrome occurs with abrupt cessation of SSRIs and SNRIs, particularly those with shorter half-lives (paroxetine, venlafaxine). Symptoms include dizziness, nausea, electric shock sensations ("brain zaps"), irritability, and insomnia. Prevention requires gradual taper over 2-4 weeks minimum, with slower tapers for longer treatment durations and higher doses (Horowitz & Taylor, 2019).

5.6 Key Takeaways

Major depressive disorder treatment proceeds from diagnostic confirmation (with specifier identification and bipolar screening) through first-line SSRI/SNRI selection matched to symptom profile, to augmentation for partial response, to treatment-resistant pathways including esketamine, Auvelity, and MAOIs. Monitoring with PHQ-9 at defined intervals provides objective data for prescribing decisions. Maintenance duration scales with episode recurrence. Discontinuation syndrome is preventable with appropriate tapering.

Chapter 6.0: Bipolar Spectrum Disorders

Bipolar disorder is the diagnosis most consequential to miss, because the treatment for unipolar depression (antidepressant monotherapy) can destabilize the illness. Every prescriber writing antidepressants has an obligation to screen for bipolarity before the first prescription. This chapter provides the prescribing framework for bipolar I, bipolar II, and cyclothymic disorder across acute mania, bipolar depression, and maintenance phases.

6.1 Diagnostic Clarification

The prescribing implications of bipolar I versus bipolar II are significant. Bipolar I requires a documented manic episode. Bipolar II requires hypomanic episodes with major depressive episodes, and patients typically spend far more time depressed than hypomanic. Cyclothymic disorder involves chronic mood fluctuation that does not meet full criteria for either mania or depression (American Psychiatric Association, 2022).

Misdiagnosis of bipolar depression as unipolar depression is common because patients seek treatment during depressive episodes and may not recognize hypomania as pathological. Features that increase bipolar suspicion include: early age of onset (teens or twenties), family history of bipolar disorder, atypical depressive features (hypersomnia, hyperphagia), psychotic features during depression, antidepressant-induced mania or rapid cycling, and multiple antidepressant failures. The MDQ screens efficiently, but a positive screen requires clinical follow-up because the MDQ's positive predictive value is limited in community samples (Hirschfeld et al., 2000).

6.2 Acute Mania Treatment

Lithium remains the gold standard for acute mania with the strongest long-term evidence for relapse prevention and unique anti-suicidal properties. Acute dosing targets levels of 0.8-1.2 mEq/L, typically requiring 900-1800mg daily in divided doses. Levels are checked 5-7 days after each dose change. Monitoring includes renal function, thyroid, calcium, and ECG at baseline with periodic reassessment (as detailed in section 4.2). The onset of antimanic effect takes 7-14 days, so adjunctive treatment is often needed acutely (Malhi et al., 2017).

Valproate (divalproex) can be initiated with a loading strategy (20-30 mg/kg/day) for rapid symptom control, targeting levels of 85-125 mcg/mL for acute mania. It is particularly effective for mixed features and rapid cycling. The teratogenicity profile makes it contraindicated in women of reproductive age unless alternatives have failed and reliable contraception is established (Stahl, 2021).

Atypical antipsychotics for acute mania include aripiprazole, quetiapine, risperidone, olanzapine, ziprasidone, asenapine, and cariprazine. Selection is guided by the side effect matrix from section 10.2. **Iloperidone (Fanapt)** received expanded FDA indication for manic and mixed episodes of bipolar I in 2024, adding another option with a relatively favorable EPS profile but requiring slow titration due to orthostatic hypotension risk (Stahl, 2021).

Consider the case of Carlos (composite example), a 28-year-old male presenting to the emergency department with pressured speech, grandiosity, decreased need for sleep (2-3 hours nightly for 5 days), impulsive spending, and irritability. His BMI is 24 and metabolic labs are normal. He has no prior psychiatric history. For first-episode mania with favorable metabolic baseline, lithium is initiated at 600mg twice daily with concurrent lorazepam 1-2mg as needed for acute agitation. An atypical antipsychotic (aripiprazole 15mg) is added for rapid symptom control while lithium reaches therapeutic levels. The plan includes lithium level check in 5 days, renal and thyroid baseline labs, and follow-up within one week of discharge.

6.3 Bipolar Depression

Bipolar depression is the predominant illness phase and the most difficult to treat. Standard antidepressant monotherapy is not recommended due to risks of mood destabilization.

Quetiapine and quetiapine XR (300mg target) have the strongest evidence for acute bipolar depression across both bipolar I and II. Sedation and metabolic effects are the primary limitations. **Lurasidone (Latuda)** at 20-120mg has FDA approval for bipolar I depression with a favorable metabolic profile, but it requires administration with food (at least 350 calories). **Cariprazine (Vraylar)** at 1.5-3mg is approved for bipolar I depression with a D3-preferring partial agonist profile. **Lumateperone (Caplyta)** at 42mg has approval for bipolar I and II depressive episodes as monotherapy or adjunctive to lithium or valproate (Calabrese et al., 2005; Stahl, 2021).

Lamotrigine is the cornerstone of bipolar depression prevention rather than acute treatment. Its slow titration schedule (25mg daily for 2 weeks, then 50mg for 2 weeks, then 100mg for 1 week, target 200mg) limits its utility for acute episodes. With concurrent valproate, the titration must be halved due to impaired glucuronidation. Stevens-Johnson syndrome risk (approximately 0.08% with proper titration) mandates strict adherence to the titration protocol (Stahl, 2021).

The antidepressant question in bipolar depression remains contentious. Guidelines generally permit short-term antidepressant use only in combination with a mood stabilizer, only for bipolar I depression refractory to first-line options, and never in patients with mixed features or a history of antidepressant-induced mania.

Bupropion and SSRIs carry lower switching risk than SNRIs and TCAs (Sachs et al., 2007).

6.4 Maintenance Treatment

Lithium is the best-studied maintenance agent with demonstrated efficacy against both manic and depressive recurrence and anti-suicidal properties. Maintenance levels target 0.6-0.8 mEq/L. Lamotrigine is preferred when the illness course is depression-predominant. Valproate is preferred when the illness course is mania-predominant. Atypical antipsychotics (aripiprazole, quetiapine, olanzapine) are maintenance options with varying metabolic trade-offs (Yatham et al., 2018).

Long-acting injectable antipsychotics are increasingly used in bipolar maintenance when adherence is a concern. **UZEDY (risperidone)** extended-release injectable received expanded indication for bipolar I maintenance in 2025, providing monthly administration options (Stahl, 2021).

6.5 Clinical Implications

Bipolar disorder prescribing requires diagnostic precision (bipolar I vs. II, current episode polarity, specifiers), phase-specific treatment selection (acute mania vs. bipolar depression vs. maintenance), teratogenicity awareness in reproductive-age patients (valproate contraindicated, lamotrigine preferred in pregnancy), and long-term monitoring commitments for mood stabilizers. The cross-reference to section 18.2 addresses perinatal bipolar management in detail.

Chapter 7.0: Anxiety Disorders

Anxiety disorders are the most common psychiatric conditions you will treat, and the pharmacological approach differs meaningfully across subtypes. Generalized anxiety, panic disorder, and social anxiety share first-line SSRI/SNRI treatment, but second-line options, PRN strategies, and augmentation approaches diverge. This chapter addresses each subtype and devotes a full section to the 2025 benzodiazepine tapering guidelines that every prescriber must know.

7.1 Generalized Anxiety Disorder

SSRIs (sertraline, escitalopram, paroxetine) and SNRIs (venlafaxine XR, duloxetine) are first-line for GAD with Level A evidence. Onset of anxiolytic effect takes 2-4 weeks. Track response with GAD-7 scores at each visit (Bandelow et al., 2017).

Buspirone (15-60mg daily in divided doses) is a 5-HT1A partial agonist with no sedation, no dependence potential, and no cognitive impairment. Its delayed onset (2-4 weeks) makes it unsuitable for acute anxiety, but as maintenance monotherapy or augmentation to an SSRI, it offers a clean side effect profile. **Hydroxyzine** (25-100mg as needed) provides short-term anxiolytic relief through H1 antagonism without dependence risk. **Gabapentin** (300-1800mg daily) and **pregabalin** (150-600mg daily) have off-label evidence for GAD, with pregabalin approved for GAD in Europe but not the US. Sedation and dizziness are the primary limitations (Stahl, 2021).

Mirtazapine (15-45mg) addresses GAD with comorbid insomnia through H1 antagonism and 5-HT2A/2C blockade. Benzodiazepines should be reserved for short-term bridge therapy (2-4 weeks maximum) while waiting for SSRI/SNRI onset. If a benzodiazepine is used, establish the taper plan before the first prescription (Bandelow et al., 2017).

7.2 Panic Disorder

SSRIs are first-line. The critical prescribing point: start at half the typical depression dose because patients with panic disorder are exquisitely sensitive to activation side effects. Sertraline: start 25mg. Escitalopram: start 5mg. Fluoxetine: start 10mg. Titrate upward slowly over 1-2 weeks (American Psychiatric Association, 2009).

Clonazepam (0.5-2mg daily) provides rapid panic suppression while the SSRI takes effect. Its longer half-life produces less interdose rebound than alprazolam. If initiated, begin taper planning at the 4-week mark. **TCAs** (imipramine, clomipramine) are effective second-line options for refractory panic but carry cardiac risks and overdose lethality.

Consider the case of Lucia (composite example), a 33-year-old woman with panic disorder presenting with 3-4 panic attacks weekly, significant anticipatory anxiety, and developing agoraphobic avoidance. She has avoided driving on highways for two months. She tried citalopram 20mg one year ago but discontinued after three days due to increased anxiety. The history of early activation on an SSRI is classic for panic disorder. The plan: start escitalopram at 5mg (below the activating threshold), titrate to 10mg at week 2, then 20mg at week 4 based on response. Concurrent clonazepam 0.25mg twice daily for 4 weeks bridges the SSRI onset period. CBT referral is placed simultaneously. The combined pharmacotherapy and psychotherapy approach has the strongest evidence for panic disorder.

7.3 Social Anxiety Disorder

SSRIs (sertraline, paroxetine, fluvoxamine) and SNRIs (venlafaxine XR) are first-line for generalized social anxiety disorder. Doses required for social anxiety tend to be at the higher end of the therapeutic range (Stein et al., 2010).

For **performance-only subtype** (stage fright, public speaking anxiety without broader social impairment), **propranolol** (10-40mg taken 30-60 minutes before performance) is the targeted treatment. It blocks peripheral beta-adrenergic symptoms (tachycardia, tremor, sweating) without affecting cognitive function. Propranolol is not effective for generalized social anxiety and should not be used as maintenance treatment. **Gabapentin** (900-3600mg daily) has supporting evidence for social anxiety and may be useful when SSRIs are insufficient (Stahl, 2021).

7.4 Benzodiazepine Management

The 2025 Joint Clinical Practice Guideline on Benzodiazepine Tapering, developed by ten medical and professional societies led by ASAM, represents the most authoritative guidance on this topic to date. Key principles follow (Brunner et al., 2025).

Risk-benefit reassessment should occur every three months for every patient on a benzodiazepine. Nearly all patients prescribed benzodiazepines for more than one month will develop physical dependence, though only approximately 1.5% develop a substance use disorder from benzodiazepine use. Physical dependence is an expected biological outcome, not a moral failing.

Tapering protocol: Initial dose reductions of 5-10% every 2-4 weeks, not exceeding 25% every 2 weeks. Patients on lower doses for shorter periods (less than 3 months) may taper faster. **Hyperbolic tapering** (progressively smaller absolute dose reductions as the total dose decreases) is recommended for the final stages of the taper, because the relationship between dose and receptor occupancy is not linear. A reduction from 2mg to 1.5mg of clonazepam does not feel the same as a reduction from 0.5mg to 0mg.

Adjunctive supports during taper include CBT, CBT-I for insomnia, hydroxyzine, gabapentin, and concurrent treatment of the underlying condition for which the benzodiazepine was prescribed. The guideline explicitly states that clinicians should not discontinue benzodiazepines abruptly in physically dependent patients and should not force tapers when patients are experiencing significant withdrawal despite gradual reduction (Brunner et al., 2025).

Equivalency conversions (see Appendix B for full table): Diazepam 10mg is approximately equivalent to alprazolam 0.5mg, clonazepam 0.5mg, and lorazepam 1mg. Converting to a longer-acting agent (diazepam or clonazepam) before tapering can smooth withdrawal symptoms for patients on short-acting benzodiazepines.

7.5 Summary and Recommendations

Anxiety disorders share SSRI/SNRI first-line treatment but diverge in second-line options and acute management strategies. Panic disorder requires low starting doses. Social anxiety may require higher-than-depression SSRI doses. Benzodiazepines serve a limited, time-defined role with mandatory taper planning from the outset. The 2025 tapering guidelines provide evidence-based structure for the deprescribing conversations that every anxious patient on chronic benzodiazepines deserves.

Chapter 8.0: Obsessive Compulsive Spectrum

OCD pharmacotherapy differs from depression treatment in two fundamental ways: higher doses are required, and longer trial durations are necessary. The prescriber who treats OCD with standard antidepressant dosing for standard antidepressant durations will conclude incorrectly that the medication failed.

8.1 OCD Pharmacotherapy

Serotonin reuptake inhibitors (SRIs) at OCD-range doses are first-line: fluoxetine 40-80mg, fluvoxamine 200-300mg, sertraline 150-200mg, paroxetine 40-60mg, escitalopram 20-40mg, citalopram 40mg. These doses are substantially higher than depression targets. An adequate OCD trial requires 8-12 weeks at maximum tolerated dose, compared to 6-8 weeks for depression (Skapinakis et al., 2016).

Clomipramine (150-250mg) remains the most potent SRI for OCD based on meta-analytic data. However, cardiac monitoring (ECG), anticholinergic side effects, and overdose lethality place it as second-line after SSRI failure. Therapeutic drug monitoring is recommended given CYP2D6-dependent metabolism.

Augmentation strategies for partial SRI response include low-dose atypical antipsychotics. Aripiprazole (2-10mg) and risperidone (0.5-2mg) have the strongest augmentation evidence. Augmentation is warranted when the patient has achieved 25-35% symptom reduction (as measured by the Yale-Brown Obsessive Compulsive Scale) after an adequate SRI trial but remains significantly impaired (Bloch et al., 2006).

Glutamate modulators represent emerging augmentation options. Memantine (5-20mg) and N-acetylcysteine (1200-2400mg) have preliminary evidence for SRI augmentation in treatment-resistant OCD, though data remain limited (Pittenger et al., 2011).

Consider the case of Andre (identifying details changed), a 38-year-old man with contamination-focused OCD who has been on sertraline 100mg for 6 weeks with minimal improvement. Before escalating treatment, the prescriber recognizes two problems: the dose is below OCD therapeutic range, and the trial duration is insufficient. Sertraline is increased to 200mg and the trial extended to 12 weeks total. At week 12, Y-BOCS scores have decreased by 30% (from 28 to 20), indicating partial response. Low-dose aripiprazole (5mg) is added as augmentation. Concurrent ERP therapy is reinforced. This sequence (optimize dose, extend duration, then augment) prevents premature treatment changes.

8.2 Related Disorders

Body dysmorphic disorder responds to SRI treatment at OCD-range doses. Antipsychotic augmentation parallels the OCD approach for partial responders. **Trichotillomania and excoriation disorder** have more limited pharmacological evidence. N-acetylcysteine (1200-2400mg daily) has the strongest data for hair-pulling, with a positive randomized controlled trial demonstrating superiority over placebo (Grant et al., 2009). SRIs may help some patients. Naltrexone (50mg) has preliminary evidence for impulse-control aspects. **Hoarding disorder** is the least responsive to pharmacotherapy within the OCD spectrum, with SRIs showing modest benefit at best.

8.3 Concluding Thoughts

OCD requires higher SRI doses, longer trial durations, and different augmentation strategies than depression. Clomipramine is the most potent SRI but carries greater risk. Atypical antipsychotic augmentation at low doses helps partial responders. N-acetylcysteine is a low-risk augmentation option for OCD-spectrum conditions involving repetitive behaviors.

Chapter 9.0: Trauma Related Disorders

PTSD pharmacotherapy has a distinct prescribing logic that differs from depression and anxiety treatment. The 2024-2025 update from the Psychopharmacology Algorithm Project at Harvard South Shore provides the most current evidence-based framework, and this chapter translates that algorithm into clinical action.

9.1 PTSD Pharmacotherapy

The algorithm begins with **sleep disturbances as the first pharmacological target**, a sequencing decision that many prescribers overlook. Trauma-related nightmares and disturbed sleep impair daytime functioning and reduce the efficacy of psychotherapy. Treating sleep first creates a foundation for subsequent interventions (Bajor et al., 2025).

Prazosin is the first-line treatment for PTSD-related nightmares and sleep disturbance. Starting dose is 1mg at bedtime, titrated by 1-2mg every 3-7 days as tolerated, with most patients responding between 5-15mg. Some patients require and tolerate doses as high as 30-45mg at bedtime. An underrecognized finding: prazosin also demonstrates efficacy for daytime PTSD symptoms, not just nightmares. The VA Practice Guideline recommended prazosin for nightmares but did not fully account for smaller controlled studies supporting its broader PTSD utility (Bajor et al., 2025).

After addressing sleep, the algorithm targets **daytime PTSD symptoms** with SSRIs. **Sertraline** and **paroxetine** are the only FDA-approved medications for PTSD. **Venlafaxine XR** has strong evidence supporting its efficacy and is recommended as an alternative first-line option. Adequate SSRI trials for PTSD require 8-12 weeks at therapeutic doses (Friedman et al., 2014).

Critical prescribing point: Benzodiazepines are ineffective for core PTSD symptoms and may increase the risk of depression and aggression. The 2025 benzodiazepine tapering guidelines (see section 7.4) strongly recommend considering benzodiazepine taper in PTSD patients. This represents a clear departure from older prescribing patterns that used benzodiazepines for PTSD-related anxiety (Bajor et al., 2025).

Consider the case of Marcus (composite example), a 41-year-old combat veteran presenting with nightly combat-related nightmares, hypervigilance, emotional numbing, and avoidance of crowded places. His PCL-5 score is 52. He currently takes alprazolam 1mg twice daily prescribed by a previous provider, which he reports "takes the edge off" but has not reduced his nightmares or hypervigilance. The prescribing plan addresses multiple targets: (1) Initiate prazosin 1mg at bedtime, titrate weekly to effect for nightmares. (2) Start sertraline 50mg daily, titrate to 150-200mg over 4 weeks. (3) Begin alprazolam taper per 2025 guidelines (5-10% reduction every 2-4 weeks) after sertraline reaches therapeutic dose. (4) Refer for prolonged exposure or CPT therapy. The sequencing matters: stabilize sleep, establish an effective SSRI, then address benzodiazepine dependence with adjunctive support.

9.2 Augmentation and Resistant PTSD

For partial SSRI response, atypical antipsychotic augmentation with quetiapine (50-300mg) or risperidone (0.5-2mg) has supporting evidence. **Pimavanserin**, a selective 5-HT2A inverse agonist, is discussed in the 2025 algorithm update as an emerging adjunctive agent for PTSD with psychotic features, with early studies suggesting benefits for sleep and distress reduction (Bajor et al., 2025).

Topiramate (25-200mg) has evidence for reducing nightmares and re-experiencing symptoms as an augmentation strategy. **Divalproex** may help PTSD-related irritability and anger.

9.3 Acute Stress and Adjustment

For **acute stress disorder**, early pharmacological intervention remains controversial. Short-term sleep support with prazosin or trazodone is reasonable. Propranolol's role in secondary prevention of PTSD (by disrupting memory consolidation) has not been consistently supported in clinical trials. **Adjustment disorders** respond to brief, targeted pharmacotherapy for the predominant symptom (anxiety or depression) with planned discontinuation after the stressor resolves or adaptation occurs.

9.4 Synthesis

PTSD pharmacotherapy follows a specific sequence: sleep disturbances first (prazosin), then daytime symptoms (SSRI/SNRI), with augmentation for partial response. Benzodiazepines are contraindicated for PTSD core symptoms. The algorithm from symptom prioritization through medication selection provides a structured approach that integrates with concurrent trauma-focused psychotherapy.

Chapter 10.0: Psychotic Disorders

Antipsychotic selection is never a one-size decision. Every agent in this class produces a distinct side effect profile determined by its receptor binding characteristics (as discussed in section 1.1), and matching the medication to the patient's risk factors is the clinical skill that separates competent prescribing from reflexive prescribing.

10.1 First Episode Psychosis

First-episode psychosis (FEP) patients respond to lower antipsychotic doses than chronically ill patients, and they are more sensitive to side effects. Starting doses should be approximately half of what chronic schizophrenia requires. Metabolic risk stratification before selection is essential: a 20-year-old presenting with FEP and a BMI of 30 should not receive olanzapine as first-line regardless of its efficacy (Correll et al., 2011).

Preferred first-line agents for FEP include aripiprazole (10-15mg), risperidone (1-3mg), or paliperidone (3-6mg). These balance efficacy with more manageable metabolic profiles compared to olanzapine or quetiapine. Duration of treatment for FEP is debated: current guidelines suggest maintaining antipsychotic treatment for at least 1-2 years following first-episode remission, with careful dose reduction considered thereafter under close monitoring (Correll et al., 2011).

10.2 Antipsychotic Selection Matrix

The selection matrix organizes antipsychotics by their principal side effect risks, enabling patient-specific prescribing:

Weight gain risk (highest to lowest): olanzapine, clozapine > quetiapine > risperidone, paliperidone > aripiprazole, ziprasidone, lurasidone, cariprazine, brexpiprazole.

EPS risk (highest to lowest): haloperidol > risperidone, paliperidone > aripiprazole, brexpiprazole > lurasidone > quetiapine, clozapine (lowest).

Prolactin elevation (highest to lowest): paliperidone, risperidone > haloperidol > olanzapine > aripiprazole, cariprazine, quetiapine (minimal to none).

QTc prolongation risk: ziprasidone, thioridazine, IV haloperidol carry the highest risk. Baseline ECG is indicated for these agents.

Cobenfy (xanomeline/trospium), approved in September 2024, represents the first antipsychotic with a fundamentally novel mechanism in decades. It acts as a muscarinic M1/M4 agonist rather than a dopamine antagonist. Trospium (a peripheral muscarinic antagonist that does not cross the blood-brain barrier) is included to mitigate peripheral cholinergic side effects. Cobenfy carries no black box warning and demonstrates a favorable metabolic, EPS, and prolactin profile compared to dopamine-blocking antipsychotics. GI side effects (nausea, constipation, dyspepsia) are the primary tolerability concerns. Clinical positioning: consider for patients with significant metabolic risk or EPS sensitivity who require antipsychotic treatment (Kaul et al., 2024).

10.3 Treatment Resistant Schizophrenia

Clozapine remains the gold standard for treatment-resistant schizophrenia (TRS), defined as failure to achieve adequate response to two antipsychotic trials of different classes at adequate doses for adequate duration (6-8 weeks each). Despite robust efficacy evidence, clozapine remains dramatically underutilized.

The **2025 elimination of the Clozapine REMS** program represents a historic change in clozapine access. The FDA determined that the REMS was no longer necessary to ensure benefits outweigh the risk of severe neutropenia. Prescribers and pharmacies are no longer required to enroll patients in a centralized database or obtain dispense authorization before each fill. However, the risk of severe neutropenia persists, and ANC monitoring remains clinically required: baseline ANC of 1500/mcL or greater (1000/mcL for patients with benign ethnic neutropenia), weekly for 6 months, biweekly for months 6-12, monthly thereafter (Stahl, 2021).

Clozapine titration starts at 12.5mg once or twice daily, increasing by 25-50mg daily as tolerated. Target dose is typically 300-450mg daily, guided by clinical response and clozapine levels (target: 350-420 ng/mL). Smoking status profoundly affects levels through CYP1A2 induction.

Consider the case of Fatima (composite example), a 29-year-old woman with schizophrenia who has failed adequate trials of aripiprazole 20mg (8 weeks), risperidone 6mg (8 weeks), and olanzapine 20mg (10 weeks, discontinued due to 25-pound weight gain). Her PANSS total score remains 95. She is a non-smoker with no history of seizures. She meets criteria for TRS. Clozapine is initiated at 12.5mg at bedtime. Baseline labs: ANC 3200/mcL, fasting glucose 92, lipid panel normal. The plan: titrate by 25mg every 2-3 days to target dose of 300mg, check clozapine level at steady state, weekly ANC for 6 months. She is counseled about reportable symptoms (fever, sore throat, flu-like illness suggesting agranulocytosis; constipation management; weight monitoring). The 2025 REMS elimination makes this initiation administratively simpler, but clinical vigilance remains unchanged.

10.4 Managing Side Effects

Tardive dyskinesia (TD) treatment has been revolutionized by VMAT2 inhibitors. **Valbenazine (Ingrezza)** at 40-80mg daily is FDA-approved for TD, with **Ingrezza Sprinkle** providing a new formulation for patients with dysphagia (2024 approval). **Deutetrabenazine (Austedo)** at 12-48mg daily (divided doses) is also FDA-approved, with CYP2D6 poor metabolizer status requiring dose reduction. Both agents reduce involuntary movements by depleting presynaptic dopamine (Stahl, 2021).

Metabolic syndrome prevention includes baseline and serial metabolic monitoring (section 4.2), lifestyle counseling, and medication selection that minimizes risk. **Metformin** (500-2000mg daily) has evidence for attenuating antipsychotic-induced weight gain when initiated concurrently or early in treatment. **Akathisia** management includes dose reduction, switching to a lower-EPS agent, propranolol (20-80mg daily), or benzodiazepines. **NMS** is a medical emergency requiring immediate antipsychotic discontinuation, dantrolene, bromocriptine, and supportive care.

10.5 Chapter Conclusions

Antipsychotic selection requires matching the medication's receptor profile to the patient's metabolic, neurological, and endocrine risk factors. Cobenfy offers the first non-dopaminergic mechanism in antipsychotic prescribing. Clozapine remains the definitive treatment for TRS, with the 2025 REMS elimination reducing access barriers while maintaining the need for clinical monitoring. VMAT2 inhibitors have transformed TD treatment.

Chapter 11.0: ADHD Across the Lifespan

ADHD prescribing carries regulatory complexity that no other diagnostic category matches. Stimulant medications are Schedule II controlled substances requiring specific prescribing practices, PDMP checks, and ongoing documentation of medical necessity. Beyond the regulatory framework, ADHD medication selection requires careful comorbidity screening, because untreated anxiety, unrecognized bipolar disorder, or active substance use disorder fundamentally changes the prescribing approach.

11.1 Assessment Before Prescribing

Before writing a stimulant prescription, screen for comorbidities that change the treatment plan. Anxiety comorbidity (present in 25-50% of adults with ADHD) may warrant starting with a non-stimulant or initiating an SSRI concurrently. Bipolar comorbidity requires mood stabilization before stimulant initiation; stimulants can precipitate mania in unstabilized bipolar disorder. Substance use disorder history shifts the risk-benefit analysis toward non-stimulants or lisdexamfetamine (with its lower misuse potential). Cardiac screening with personal and family cardiac history is required before stimulant initiation; baseline ECG is recommended when cardiac risk factors are present (Kooij et al., 2019).

11.2 Stimulant Medications

Methylphenidate formulations differ primarily in delivery mechanism and duration of action. Immediate-release (Ritalin) lasts 3-4 hours. Extended-release formulations include Concerta (osmotic release, 10-12 hours), Ritalin LA (bead technology, 6-8 hours), Aptensio XR (8-12 hours), and Jornay PM (evening dosing for morning effect). Starting dose for adults: 10-20mg daily IR or equivalent ER, titrating by 10-20mg weekly to response (Stahl, 2021).

Amphetamine formulations include mixed amphetamine salts IR (Adderall, 4-6 hours) and XR (Adderall XR, 10-12 hours), lisdexamfetamine (Vyvanse, prodrug with 12-14 hour duration), and dextroamphetamine (Dexedrine). Lisdexamfetamine's prodrug design requires enzymatic conversion in the bloodstream, producing a smoother onset curve and lower abuse potential than immediate-release amphetamines. Starting dose for adults: 20mg XR formulation, titrating by 10-20mg weekly (Stahl, 2021).

Head-to-head, methylphenidate and amphetamine are comparably effective at the population level. Individual response varies: approximately 70% of patients respond to the first stimulant tried, and an additional 15-20% respond when switched to the other class. If a patient does not respond to adequate methylphenidate, try amphetamine before concluding stimulant failure (Faraone, 2018).

The **2025 FDA class-wide ER stimulant label update** adds a clearer limitation-of-use signal for children under 6 years, reflecting higher plasma exposure and rates of adverse effects (including clinically significant weight loss) in this age group. This does not constitute a contraindication but reinforces that behavioral interventions should be attempted first in preschool-aged children (FDA, 2025).

Consider the case of Amanda (composite example), a 32-year-old woman diagnosed with ADHD (combined presentation) who also has GAD managed with sertraline 100mg. She reports that sertraline has controlled her anxiety well, but she continues to struggle with organization, task initiation, and sustained attention at work. Her ASRS screening score is 16. Given her concurrent anxiety management with an SSRI, a stimulant can be initiated concurrently. Lisdexamfetamine 30mg is chosen for its smooth onset profile (less likely to spike anxiety than IR formulations) and its once-daily dosing. She is counseled about potential anxiety reactivation and instructed to contact the clinic if anxiety worsens before the next scheduled visit in 4 weeks.

11.3 Non-Stimulant Options

Atomoxetine (40-100mg daily) is a selective norepinephrine reuptake inhibitor with no abuse potential. It is metabolized by CYP2D6; poor metabolizers achieve higher levels and require dose reduction (as discussed in section 3.2). Onset of full effect takes 4-6 weeks. It is particularly useful in ADHD with comorbid anxiety or substance use disorder (Stahl, 2021).

Viloxazine ER (Qelbree) is a newer norepinephrine reuptake inhibitor approved for ADHD in children, adolescents, and adults. Adult dosing: 200-600mg daily. It has a distinct mechanism from atomoxetine with additional serotonergic modulation. **Alpha-2 agonists** include guanfacine ER (Intuniv, 1-4mg daily) and clonidine ER (Kapvay, 0.1-0.4mg daily). These agents are particularly useful for ADHD with comorbid tic disorders, aggression, or oppositional behavior. **Onyda XR (clonidine)**, a new liquid suspension formulation approved in 2024, expands options for pediatric patients who cannot swallow tablets (Stahl, 2021).

11.4 Complex Presentations

ADHD + anxiety: Start the SSRI/SNRI, stabilize anxiety, then add the stimulant. Or start a non-stimulant (atomoxetine) that addresses both. **ADHD + bipolar**: Stabilize mood first with lithium, valproate, or an atypical antipsychotic. Only then introduce a stimulant cautiously at low dose with close monitoring for mood destabilization. **ADHD + substance use disorder**: Prefer lisdexamfetamine (lower misuse potential) or non-stimulants. Avoid immediate-release stimulants. Monitor for diversion. **ADHD + tic disorders**: Alpha-2 agonists as first-line. Stimulants can be used cautiously (they do not cause tics in most patients, despite historical concerns). **ADHD +**

autism: Lower starting doses, slower titration, and heightened side effect monitoring (Kooij et al., 2019).

11.5 Essential Points

ADHD prescribing requires comorbidity screening before medication selection. Stimulants are first-line for uncomplicated ADHD. If one stimulant class fails, try the other before concluding stimulant failure. Non-stimulants serve patients with comorbid anxiety, substance use disorders, or tic disorders. Complex presentations require sequential treatment: stabilize the comorbid condition first, then address ADHD.

Chapter 12.0: Sleep and Insomnia Disorders

Sleep disruption is the most common symptom you will encounter across every psychiatric diagnosis. It is also the symptom patients most urgently want addressed. The temptation to prescribe a benzodiazepine or Z-drug at the first visit is strong, and it is almost always the wrong long-term strategy. This chapter provides the evidence-based pharmacological hierarchy for insomnia that prioritizes safety, avoids dependence, and matches mechanism to the patient's specific sleep disturbance.

12.1 Insomnia Pharmacotherapy

CBT-I (cognitive behavioral therapy for insomnia) remains the first-line treatment with long-term efficacy exceeding pharmacotherapy. When medication is needed, the selection depends on the type of insomnia and the patient's risk factors (Qaseem et al., 2016).

Orexin receptor antagonists (DORAs) represent the preferred pharmacological class for chronic insomnia. **Suvorexant (Belsomra)** at 10-20mg and **lemborexant (Dayvigo)** at 5-10mg block orexin-mediated wakefulness without potentiating GABA, avoiding the dependence and cognitive impairment associated with older agents. They are effective for both sleep onset and sleep maintenance. Daytime somnolence is the primary side effect (Herring et al., 2012).

Ramelteon (Rozerem) is a melatonin MT1/MT2 receptor agonist at 8mg nightly. It specifically targets sleep onset without affecting sleep architecture or producing next-day sedation. No abuse potential, no dependence, no rebound insomnia. Useful in elderly patients where cognitive safety is paramount.

Low-dose doxepin (Silenor) at 3-6mg is FDA-approved specifically for sleep maintenance insomnia through selective H1 antagonism at these ultra-low doses. It does not produce the antidepressant effects or anticholinergic burden seen at antidepressant doses (25-300mg). **Trazodone** (25-100mg) is the most commonly prescribed off-label sleep medication. It produces sedation through 5-HT2A antagonism and H1 blockade. Priapism is a rare but serious risk requiring patient education. **Gabapentin** (100-600mg) is useful for insomnia with comorbid pain or anxiety (Stahl, 2021).

Z-drugs (zolpidem, zaleplon, eszopiclone) carry a black box warning for complex sleep behaviors (sleep-driving, sleep-eating, sleep-walking). They are appropriate for short-term use (2-4 weeks) but not chronic insomnia management. Tolerance develops, and discontinuation produces rebound insomnia. In the elderly, fall risk and cognitive effects make Z-drugs particularly problematic (Qaseem et al., 2016).

Consider the case of Robert (composite example), a 68-year-old man with insomnia presenting with difficulty maintaining sleep (wakes at 2 AM nightly and cannot return to sleep). He takes lisinopril and atorvastatin. His previous provider prescribed zolpidem 10mg, which he has taken nightly for three years. He wants to "get off the sleeping pill." The plan addresses both the insomnia and the Z-drug dependence: (1) Start lemborexant 5mg nightly (targeting the underlying insomnia with a non-GABA mechanism). (2) Begin gradual zolpidem taper over 8-12 weeks (reducing by 25% every 2-3 weeks). (3) Refer for CBT-I to build sustainable sleep behaviors. (4) If sleep maintenance insomnia persists despite lemborexant, add low-dose doxepin 3mg for its targeted H1 mechanism. The pharmacological logic matches the sleep disturbance type while removing the agent with dependence risk.

12.2 Medication Induced Sleep Issues

SSRI/SNRI activation can disrupt sleep, especially in the first 2-4 weeks. Management options include taking the medication in the morning, adding trazodone 25-50mg at bedtime, or switching to a less activating agent. Stimulant-related insomnia is managed by timing the last dose before 2 PM for IR formulations or switching to shorter-duration ER formulations. Antipsychotic sedation that impairs daytime functioning is managed by shifting the full dose to bedtime or switching to a less sedating agent (Stahl, 2021).

12.3 Chapter Overview

Insomnia pharmacotherapy follows a hierarchy: CBT-I first, then DORAs or ramelteon for chronic insomnia, low-dose doxepin for sleep maintenance, trazodone for comorbid situations, and Z-drugs or benzodiazepines only for short-term use with a built-in exit strategy. Elderly patients require particular attention to fall risk, cognitive effects, and anticholinergic burden.

Chapter 13.0: Substance Use Disorders

Substance use disorders are pharmacologically treatable conditions, and underprescribing of evidence-based medications remains a far greater clinical problem than overprescribing. Fewer than 20% of patients with alcohol use disorder and fewer than 35% of patients with opioid use disorder receive any medication treatment. This chapter covers the FDA-approved pharmacotherapies and their clinical application.

13.1 Alcohol Use Disorder

Naltrexone (oral 50mg daily or injectable 380mg monthly as Vivitrol) is first-line for AUD. It blocks mu-opioid receptors, reducing the reinforcing effects of alcohol and decreasing heavy drinking days. The injectable formulation eliminates adherence variability. Contraindications: current opioid use (precipitates withdrawal), acute hepatitis. LFTs should be monitored at baseline and periodically (Jonas et al., 2014).

Acamprosate (666mg three times daily) modulates glutamate neurotransmission and is most effective in maintaining abstinence after detoxification. It is renally eliminated with no hepatic metabolism, making it the preferred choice in patients with hepatic impairment. **Disulfiram** (250mg daily) produces an aversive reaction (flushing, nausea, tachycardia) when combined with alcohol through acetaldehyde accumulation. Patient selection requires motivation and reliability; it is most effective with supervised administration (Jonas et al., 2014).

Gabapentin (600-1800mg daily) has off-label evidence for AUD, particularly in patients with concurrent insomnia and anxiety. **Topiramate** (200-300mg daily) reduces heavy drinking through glutamate modulation and GABA enhancement (Stahl, 2021).

13.2 Opioid Use Disorder

Buprenorphine/naloxone (Suboxone) is the most widely prescribed MOUD. Traditional induction requires the patient to be in mild-to-moderate withdrawal (COWS score of 8-12) before the first dose to avoid precipitated withdrawal. **Micro-induction** protocols allow overlapping buprenorphine initiation without full withdrawal, starting at 0.5mg and increasing over 3-7 days. The X-waiver requirement for prescribing buprenorphine was eliminated in 2023, allowing any DEA-registered provider to prescribe. Maintenance doses of 16-24mg daily are typical (SAMHSA, 2024).

Sublocade (buprenorphine extended-release injection) received a 2025 label update allowing rapid initiation, permitting transition to monthly injection after minimal transmucosal exposure rather than requiring a prolonged oral lead-in period. This targets the real-world attrition point where patients stabilize on oral buprenorphine but drop out before transitioning to the injectable (Stahl, 2021).

Methadone requires dispensing through an Opioid Treatment Program (OTP). It has the longest evidence base for OUD treatment. QTc monitoring is recommended, particularly above 100mg daily. **Naltrexone XR (Vivitrol)** monthly injection is effective for OUD but requires complete opioid detoxification (7-14 days) before initiation, which is the primary clinical barrier.

Consider the case of Malik (identifying details changed), a 34-year-old man with OUD who presents requesting treatment. He last used fentanyl 18 hours ago and is experiencing early withdrawal (COWS: 10). He has tried methadone previously but discontinued due to daily clinic requirements. A micro-induction protocol is initiated: buprenorphine 0.5mg sublingually, repeated in 2 hours if tolerated, increasing to 2mg by end of day one, 8mg on day two, and target 16-24mg by day three. Once stabilized on oral buprenorphine for one week, he is transitioned to Sublocade 300mg monthly injection using the rapid initiation pathway. This approach reduces the window of vulnerability between treatment initiation and sustained medication adherence.

13.3 Other Substance Disorders

Stimulant use disorder has no FDA-approved pharmacotherapy. Emerging evidence supports mirtazapine, topiramate, and bupropion/naltrexone combinations. Treatment focuses on managing comorbid conditions and providing behavioral interventions. **Cannabis use disorder**: N-acetylcysteine has positive trial data in adolescents (Gray et al., 2012). Gabapentin may reduce withdrawal symptoms. **Tobacco use disorder**: Varenicline (1mg twice daily, preceded by 1-week titration) is the most effective single agent. Bupropion SR (150mg twice daily) is the second-line pharmacotherapy. Combination NRT (patch plus lozenge or gum) approaches varenicline efficacy (Stahl, 2021).

13.4 Dual Diagnosis Prescribing

When psychiatric and substance use disorders co-occur, both conditions require concurrent treatment. Select medications that address both conditions when possible: naltrexone for AUD with comorbid depression (some evidence for mood benefit), bupropion for depression with comorbid tobacco dependence, gabapentin for anxiety with comorbid AUD. Avoid benzodiazepines in patients with any substance use disorder history. Document informed consent when prescribing controlled substances to patients with SUD (Stahl, 2021).

13.5 Integration and Application

Medication treatment for substance use disorders is evidence-based, effective, and dramatically underutilized. The prescriber's role includes overcoming personal and systemic biases against pharmacotherapy for addiction, initiating treatment at the point of clinical contact (not deferring to specialty programs that may not exist locally), and integrating SUD treatment with psychiatric medication management.

Chapter 14.0: Eating Disorder Prescribing

Pharmacotherapy for eating disorders plays a supporting role to nutritional rehabilitation and psychotherapy, not a leading one. The evidence base is limited compared to other psychiatric diagnoses, and the prescriber's primary obligation is often to avoid harm (no bupropion in purging patients, no appetite-suppressing agents in anorexia) rather than to achieve aggressive pharmacological response.

14.1 Anorexia and Bulimia

Anorexia nervosa has the weakest pharmacotherapy evidence of any eating disorder. No medication has demonstrated reliable efficacy for weight restoration or core anorexia psychopathology. Olanzapine (2.5-10mg) has modest evidence for reducing anxiety around eating and facilitating weight gain through H1 and 5-HT2C antagonism. SSRIs are generally ineffective during the acute malnourished state but may become useful for comorbid depression and anxiety after weight restoration. Bupropion is contraindicated due to seizure risk in underweight and purging patients (Attia et al., 2019).

Bulimia nervosa has a single FDA-approved medication: fluoxetine at 60mg daily. This is higher than the typical depression dose and should be titrated to the full 60mg. Other SSRIs at higher doses have supporting evidence but lack formal approval. Topiramate (25-200mg) has off-label evidence for reducing binge-purge frequency but carries weight loss effects that may be problematic in some patients. Bupropion is absolutely contraindicated in bulimia due to the elevated seizure risk associated with purging-induced electrolyte abnormalities (Stahl, 2021).

14.2 Binge Eating and ARFID

Binge eating disorder is the only eating disorder with a non-SSRI FDA-approved medication. **Lisdexamfetamine (Vyvanse)** at 50-70mg daily reduces binge frequency through dopaminergic effects on impulse control. It is not approved for weight loss and should not be prescribed for that purpose. SSRIs and SNRIs at standard antidepressant doses may help when comorbid depression is present. Topiramate has off-label evidence for binge reduction with concurrent weight loss (McElroy et al., 2016).

ARFID (avoidant/restrictive food intake disorder) has minimal pharmacotherapy evidence. Mirtazapine (7.5-30mg) may increase appetite through 5-HT2C and H1 antagonism. Cyproheptadine (4-8mg) has been used as an appetite stimulant in pediatric populations. When ARFID is driven by sensory anxiety, low-dose SSRIs may help address the anxiety component.

14.3 Clinical Implications

Eating disorder prescribing demands awareness of what medications can harm. The bupropion contraindication in purging disorders is absolute. QTc monitoring is critical in malnourished patients. Electrolyte monitoring is essential before initiating psychotropic medications in patients who purge. Medication is adjunctive to nutritional rehabilitation and structured psychotherapy, not a substitute.

Chapter 15.0: Neurocognitive Disorders

Neurocognitive disorder prescribing serves two distinct goals: slowing cognitive decline (where evidence now includes disease-modifying therapies for Alzheimer's) and managing behavioral and psychological symptoms that cause acute distress and functional impairment. The 2025 APA delirium guidelines have changed the approach to behavioral management, and this chapter integrates those updates.

15.1 Alzheimer's Pharmacotherapy

Cholinesterase inhibitors (donepezil 5-23mg, rivastigmine 3-12mg or patch 4.6-13.3mg, galantamine 8-24mg) remain the foundation of Alzheimer's treatment. They produce modest, time-limited cognitive benefits by enhancing cholinergic transmission. **Zunveyl (benzgalantamine)**, a delayed-release formulation of a galantamine precursor approved in 2024, was designed to reduce the GI side effects that limit cholinesterase inhibitor tolerability. **Memantine** (10-28mg daily), an NMDA receptor antagonist, is used alone or in combination with a cholinesterase inhibitor for moderate-to-severe Alzheimer's (Stahl, 2021).

Anti-amyloid therapies represent a paradigm shift. **Lecanemab (Leqembi)** and **donanemab (Kisunla)** are monoclonal antibodies that clear amyloid plaques and have demonstrated statistically significant (though clinically modest) slowing of cognitive decline in early symptomatic Alzheimer's. Both require amyloid PET or CSF confirmation of amyloid pathology before initiation and serial MRI monitoring for amyloid-related imaging abnormalities (ARIA), including edema and microhemorrhages. **Lumipulse**, the first FDA-cleared blood test to aid Alzheimer's diagnosis in cognitively impaired adults, was cleared in 2025, potentially simplifying the diagnostic pathway (van Dyck et al., 2023).

15.2 Behavioral Symptoms

Non-pharmacologic interventions are first-line for BPSD (behavioral and psychological symptoms of dementia): structured routines, environmental modifications, caregiver education, and addressing unmet needs (pain, constipation, infection).

Brexpiprazole (Rexulti) at 2-3mg is the only FDA-approved medication specifically for agitation associated with Alzheimer's dementia. All other antipsychotic use in dementia is off-label and carries the black box warning for increased mortality in elderly patients with dementia-related psychosis. **Citalopram** at doses up to 20mg (limited by QTc risk in elderly) demonstrated agitation reduction in the CITAD trial. Trazodone (25-150mg) may help with agitation and sundowning (Stahl, 2021).

The **2025 APA delirium guidelines** recommend against antipsychotics for delirium prevention or routine treatment. Antipsychotics should be reserved for severe agitation or distress that poses safety risks, and only after nonpharmacologic strategies and reversible contributors (medication effects, infection, metabolic derangement) have been addressed. For patients undergoing major surgery, dexmedetomidine is suggested over other sedating agents for delirium prevention (APA, 2025).

15.3 Other Dementias

Lewy body dementia patients are extremely sensitive to antipsychotic medications (severe EPS, potentially fatal reactions even at low doses). Cholinesterase inhibitors are prioritized for cognitive and behavioral symptoms. **Pimavanserin (Nuplazid)**, a selective 5-HT2A inverse agonist, is FDA-approved for Parkinson's disease psychosis and is the preferred antipsychotic agent in Lewy body/Parkinson's dementia due to its lack of dopamine blockade. **Frontotemporal dementia** shows limited response to cholinesterase inhibitors. SSRIs (sertraline, citalopram) and trazodone may help with disinhibition, compulsive behaviors, and agitation (Stahl, 2021).

15.4 Chapter Conclusions

Neurocognitive disorder prescribing now spans from symptomatic cholinesterase inhibitors through disease-modifying anti-amyloid therapies that require specialized monitoring. Behavioral symptoms warrant nonpharmacologic approaches first, with brexpiprazole as the only specifically approved agent for Alzheimer's agitation. The 2025 delirium guidelines significantly restrict antipsychotic use in delirium management.

Chapter 16.0: Personality Disorder Prescribing

Personality disorders are not primary targets for pharmacotherapy. No medication treats a personality disorder as a whole. What medication can do is target specific symptom dimensions (affective dysregulation, impulsivity, cognitive-perceptual disturbance) that cause acute distress and functional impairment. The prescriber who understands this distinction avoids the polypharmacy trap that personality disorder presentations frequently produce.

16.1 Borderline Personality Disorder

BPD pharmacotherapy is organized by symptom domain, not by the diagnosis itself (Lieb et al., 2010).

Affective dysregulation (emotional lability, depressive crashes, anger storms): Mood stabilizers are the first option. Lamotrigine (100-200mg) has evidence for reducing emotional reactivity and depressive symptoms. Valproate has evidence for impulsive aggression. SSRIs (fluoxetine, sertraline) may reduce affective instability modestly, though effect sizes are smaller than for mood stabilizers.

Impulsivity and aggression: Mood stabilizers (lamotrigine, valproate, lithium) and SSRIs have the best evidence. Low-dose atypical antipsychotics (aripiprazole 5-15mg, olanzapine 2.5-10mg) can help with impulsive aggression.

Cognitive-perceptual symptoms (transient paranoid ideation, dissociation, quasi-psychotic experiences): Low-dose atypical antipsychotics provide short-term relief. Aripiprazole and olanzapine have the most evidence.

Medications to avoid: Benzodiazepines (disinhibition risk, paradoxical aggression, dependence in a population prone to self-harm and overdose). TCAs (lethal in overdose, and BPD patients are at elevated suicide risk). **Polypharmacy avoidance** is a clinical priority: the patient with BPD on an SSRI, a mood stabilizer, an atypical antipsychotic, and a benzodiazepine is overmedicated. Each medication should have a specific target symptom and a defined trial period. If it isn't working, stop it before adding something else (Lieb et al., 2010).

Consider the case of Isabella (composite example), a 26-year-old woman with BPD presenting with severe emotional lability, self-harm (cutting on forearms, 2-3 times weekly), and impulsive spending. She is currently on fluoxetine 60mg, quetiapine 200mg, and clonazepam 1mg twice daily (prescribed by a previous provider). Her self-harm has not improved on this regimen. The prescribing reassessment identifies three problems: (1) Clonazepam carries disinhibition risk and overdose potential in a self-harming patient. (2) Quetiapine at 200mg is producing 15-pound weight gain without clear target symptom improvement. (3) Fluoxetine alone has not controlled emotional lability. The plan: taper clonazepam per 2025 guidelines (section 7.4). Reduce and discontinue quetiapine. Initiate lamotrigine (targeting affective dysregulation) with standard titration. Maintain fluoxetine. The result: fewer medications, each with a clearer rationale, and removal of agents carrying specific risks in this population.

16.2 Other Personality Disorders

Schizotypal personality disorder may benefit from low-dose atypical antipsychotics for referential thinking and social anxiety. **Avoidant personality disorder** responds to SSRIs targeting the social anxiety component. **Antisocial personality disorder** has the weakest pharmacotherapy evidence; medications address comorbid conditions (depression, substance use, impulsive aggression) rather than the personality pattern itself (Stahl, 2021).

16.3 Summary

Personality disorder prescribing is symptom-targeted, not diagnosis-targeted. Every medication must have a defined symptom target and trial period. Polypharmacy reduction is often the most therapeutic prescribing intervention. Benzodiazepines and TCAs carry specific risks in BPD populations.

Chapter 17.0: Neurodevelopmental Prescribing

Prescribing for neurodevelopmental conditions requires modified dosing strategies, heightened side effect sensitivity awareness, and respect for the fact that many psychotropic medications are used off-label in these populations. Patients with autism spectrum disorder, intellectual disability, and tic disorders often respond differently to standard psychiatric medications, and the prescriber who applies standard adult protocols without modification will produce more side effects and less benefit.

17.1 Autism Spectrum Disorder

Two medications carry FDA approval for irritability associated with ASD: **risperidone** (0.25-3mg, approved for ages 5-16) and **aripiprazole** (2-15mg, approved for ages 6-17). "Irritability" in the FDA indication encompasses aggression, self-injury, and severe tantrums, not the broader range of ASD-associated challenges (Owen et al., 2009).

SSRIs are commonly used for repetitive behaviors and comorbid anxiety in ASD, but response rates are lower and side effect rates higher than in neurotypical populations. Start at lower doses (e.g., fluoxetine 5mg) and titrate more slowly. Behavioral activation and disinhibition are more common SSRI side effects in ASD. **Alpha-2 agonists** (guanfacine, clonidine) are useful for hyperactivity and impulsivity in ASD, often better tolerated than stimulants. **Stimulants** for comorbid ADHD are effective but require lower starting doses and closer monitoring for irritability and appetite suppression. **Melatonin** (1-5mg) is first-line for the sleep initiation difficulties that affect up to 80% of children with ASD (Stahl, 2021).

Consider the case of Ravi (composite example), a 9-year-old boy with ASD (Level 2 support needs) presenting with severe aggression toward caregivers (hitting, biting) occurring 3-5 times daily, significant hyperactivity, and sleep onset taking 2-3 hours nightly. Current medications: none. The prescribing plan addresses symptoms sequentially: (1) Melatonin 3mg at bedtime for sleep onset. (2) Guanfacine ER 1mg daily for hyperactivity and impulsivity (starting low, titrating to 2-3mg over weeks). (3) If aggression persists after adequate guanfacine trial, add aripiprazole starting at 2mg daily. The rationale: sleep improvement often reduces daytime behavioral dysregulation, and guanfacine addresses hyperactivity without the metabolic risks of antipsychotics. Aripiprazole is held in reserve because metabolic monitoring is a lifelong commitment once initiated in a young patient.

17.2 Intellectual Disability

Prescribing in intellectual disability requires recognition that patients may not be able to self-report side effects. Behavioral changes may be the only signal of akathisia, constipation, or sedation. Monitoring parameters should include caregiver observation checklists, regular weight tracking, and metabolic labs at the same intervals recommended for general populations. The threshold for prescribing antipsychotics for behavioral management should be high, with documentation of behavioral interventions attempted before pharmacotherapy (Stahl, 2021).

17.3 Tic Disorders and Tourette

Alpha-2 agonists (guanfacine ER, clonidine ER) are first-line for tic disorders based on favorable risk-benefit ratios. **Atypical antipsychotics** (aripiprazole 2-10mg, risperidone 0.25-2mg) are second-line for moderate to severe tics. **VMAT2 inhibitors** (deutetrabenazine, valbenazine) have emerging evidence for tic reduction. **Ecopipam**, a novel D1 receptor antagonist, showed positive results in a 12-month open-label extension study in pediatric Tourette syndrome in 2025, representing a potential new mechanism for tic treatment that avoids D2 blockade and its associated risks (Gilbert et al., 2018; Stahl, 2021).

17.4 Synthesis

Neurodevelopmental prescribing requires lower starting doses, slower titration, heightened side effect monitoring, and sequential treatment targeting the most impairing symptoms first. Medication is adjunctive to behavioral interventions, not a substitute. The metabolic commitment of antipsychotic prescribing in young patients warrants conservative use and regular reassessment of continued need.

Part III: Special Populations and Clinical Situations

Chapters 18 through 22: Perinatal, Pediatric, Geriatric, Medical Comorbidity, Emergencies

Chapter 18.0: Perinatal Psychiatric Prescribing

The question is never simply if a medication is "safe" in pregnancy. The question is if the risk of the untreated psychiatric illness to the mother and fetus exceeds the risk of the medication. Untreated maternal depression increases preterm birth risk, low birth weight, preeclampsia, and impaired mother-infant bonding. Untreated maternal psychosis is a medical emergency. Every prescribing decision during the perinatal period is a risk-benefit calculation with two patients, and the prescriber who defaults to stopping all medications "just to be safe" is making an active treatment decision with its own consequences.

18.1 Preconception Planning

Preconception counseling is the ideal clinical scenario because it allows time for thoughtful medication transitions. The core question: is this patient on a medication with known teratogenic risk that can be replaced with a safer alternative before conception?

Valproate is the highest-priority medication to discontinue before pregnancy. Neural tube defect rates of 1-2% and neurodevelopmental effects (including reduced IQ and increased autism risk) in 30-40% of exposed pregnancies make valproate effectively contraindicated in pregnancy-capable patients unless no alternative exists (Tomson et al., 2018). Transition to **lamotrigine** (the preferred mood stabilizer in pregnancy) should occur months before conception to allow titration and mood stability confirmation.

Lithium carries teratogenic risk for Ebstein's anomaly (cardiac malformation), though the absolute risk is lower than historically believed, approximately 0.1-0.2% versus 0.005% baseline (Patorno et al., 2017). The clinical decision depends on illness severity. For patients with severe, recurrent bipolar I disorder where lithium is the only effective mood stabilizer, continuation through pregnancy with close monitoring (monthly lithium levels, fetal echocardiography at 16-20 weeks) may be more appropriate than discontinuation and relapse risk.

Carbamazepine is a known teratogen (neural tube defects, craniofacial abnormalities) and should be replaced before conception when possible. **Topiramate** carries cleft palate risk and should be discontinued. **Benzodiazepines** in the first trimester are associated with a small increased risk of cleft palate, though recent meta-analyses suggest the risk is lower than previously thought. In all cases, folic acid supplementation at 4mg daily (higher than the standard 0.4mg prenatal dose) is recommended for patients on or recently discontinued from antiepileptic medications (ACOG, 2023).

18.2 Prescribing During Pregnancy

The 2023 ACOG Clinical Practice Guideline provides the most current framework for perinatal psychiatric medication management. The guiding principle: use the lowest effective number of medications at the lowest effective dose that maintains psychiatric stability (ACOG, 2023).

Depression in pregnancy affects 10-20% of pregnant individuals. SSRIs are first-line, with **sertraline** generally preferred due to extensive safety data and low placental transfer. **Escitalopram** and **fluoxetine** also have reassuring safety profiles. The primary concerns with SSRI exposure are: neonatal adaptation syndrome (jitteriness, feeding difficulties, respiratory distress in the first few days of life, typically self-limited), a possible small increased risk of persistent pulmonary hypertension of the newborn (PPHN) with third-trimester exposure (absolute risk remains below 1%), and a modest increase in preterm birth that may reflect the underlying depression rather than the medication (Huybrechts et al., 2014).

Bupropion has a growing safety profile in pregnancy without significant teratogenicity signals. **SNRIs** (venlafaxine, duloxetine) have less extensive pregnancy data than SSRIs but no confirmed major teratogenic risks. The clinical decision between switching a stable patient from an SNRI to an SSRI for pregnancy versus maintaining the effective SNRI depends on illness severity and prior treatment history.

Anxiety in pregnancy is managed primarily with SSRIs. Benzodiazepine use during pregnancy is discouraged but not absolutely contraindicated. When used, lorazepam is often preferred because it lacks active metabolites and has a shorter half-life than diazepam. Third-trimester benzodiazepine use can produce neonatal sedation and withdrawal symptoms.

Bipolar disorder in pregnancy presents the most complex prescribing decisions. **Lamotrigine** is the preferred mood stabilizer: no confirmed teratogenicity, though levels decrease significantly during pregnancy due to increased renal clearance and hepatic glucuronidation (requiring dose increases, sometimes doubling the pre-pregnancy dose, with close monitoring). **Lithium** is an option with cardiac monitoring as described in section 18.1. Atypical antipsychotics, particularly **olanzapine** (the most studied in pregnancy) and **quetiapine**, can be used for bipolar management when mood stabilizers alone are insufficient (ACOG, 2023).

Psychosis in pregnancy requires continued antipsychotic treatment. Discontinuation risks relapse, which poses far greater risk to mother and fetus than medication exposure. Maintain the lowest effective dose and monitor for gestational diabetes (antipsychotic metabolic effects compound pregnancy-related insulin resistance).

Consider the case of Elena (composite example), a 29-year-old woman with bipolar I disorder maintained on lithium 900mg and quetiapine 200mg, now 8 weeks pregnant (unplanned). Her last manic episode occurred 14 months ago. The prescribing decision is not straightforward. Discontinuing lithium carries significant relapse risk (50% relapse rate in the first trimester after abrupt discontinuation). Continuing lithium requires informed consent, monthly lithium levels (levels decrease as renal clearance increases during pregnancy), fetal echocardiography at 16-20 weeks, and neonatal monitoring at delivery. The prescriber discusses options with Elena and her obstetrician: (1) Continue lithium with enhanced monitoring, accepting the small cardiac risk. (2) Cross-taper to lamotrigine, accepting 6-8 weeks of potential mood vulnerability during the transition. (3) Maintain quetiapine and discontinue lithium, relying on quetiapine monotherapy (less evidence for mania prevention). Elena chooses to continue lithium with monitoring. The decision is documented with informed consent, risks and benefits discussed, and multidisciplinary coordination established.

18.3 Postpartum Mental Health

The postpartum period carries the highest psychiatric risk of a woman's lifetime. Postpartum depression affects 10-20% of new mothers. Postpartum psychosis, though rare (1-2 per 1,000 births), is a psychiatric emergency requiring immediate intervention.

SSRIs are first-line for postpartum depression, with sertraline and paroxetine having the lowest breast milk transfer ratios. Standard dosing and titration apply. Two novel agents specifically target postpartum depression through neurosteroid mechanisms:

Brexanolone (Zulresso) is a synthetic allopregnanolone administered as a continuous 60-hour IV infusion in a certified healthcare facility. It produces rapid antidepressant response (within 24-48 hours) through positive allosteric modulation of GABA-A receptors. REMS requirements include continuous pulse oximetry monitoring due to sedation and syncope risk. Its use is limited by cost, IV administration requirements, and facility certification (Meltzer-Brody et al., 2018).

Zuranolone (Zurzuvae) is an oral neurosteroid (neuroactive steroid GABA-A receptor positive allosteric modulator) taken as 50mg nightly for 14 days. It provides the mechanistic advantage of neurosteroid modulation without the IV infusion and facility requirements of brexanolone. Dizziness, somnolence, and sedation are the primary side effects. Patients should not drive or operate heavy machinery for at least 12 hours after each dose (Deligiannidis et al., 2023).

Postpartum psychosis typically presents within the first 2-4 weeks postpartum with rapid onset of confusion, disorganized behavior, paranoia, hallucinations, and mood lability. It is a psychiatric emergency. Initial management includes hospitalization, safety assessment (infanticide risk must be evaluated), and pharmacotherapy with a sedating antipsychotic (olanzapine 10-20mg or haloperidol 5-10mg) combined with a benzodiazepine (lorazepam 1-2mg) for acute stabilization. Mood stabilizer initiation (lithium or valproate) follows once acute psychosis is controlled, as the majority of postpartum psychosis cases occur in the context of bipolar disorder (ACOG, 2023).

18.4 Lactation Considerations

The decision to breastfeed while taking psychiatric medication involves weighing the significant health benefits of breastfeeding against the typically small amount of medication exposure through breast milk.

Preferred medications during breastfeeding by class: For SSRIs, **sertraline** and **paroxetine** produce the lowest infant serum levels and are generally compatible with breastfeeding. For mood stabilizers, **lamotrigine** is compatible with breastfeeding with infant monitoring (serum levels in breastfed infants reach approximately 25% of maternal levels). **Lithium** is generally avoided during breastfeeding due to variable infant serum levels and the risk of dehydration-related toxicity, though clinical decisions are individualized for patients where lithium is the only effective treatment. **Valproate** is compatible with breastfeeding at relatively low transfer rates. For antipsychotics, **olanzapine** and **quetiapine** have the most reassuring lactation data (Stahl, 2021).

Key resources for real-time lactation safety decisions include **LactMed** (National Library of Medicine database, free and regularly updated), **InfantRisk** (provider consultation service from Texas Tech University), and **MotherToBaby** (patient-facing fact sheets).

Consider the case of Jasmine (identifying details changed), a 34-year-old woman with recurrent MDD who delivered 3 weeks ago and is now presenting with PHQ-9 of 21, severe insomnia despite infant sleeping 4-hour stretches, intrusive thoughts of harming her baby (ego-dystonic, no intent or plan), and significant guilt. She is breastfeeding and does not want to stop. The clinical assessment distinguishes postpartum depression with intrusive thoughts (common, ego-dystonic, not associated with intent) from postpartum psychosis (disorganization, loss of reality testing). Her presentation is consistent with severe postpartum depression. Treatment: sertraline 50mg (compatible with breastfeeding), titrating to 100mg at 2 weeks. For the severe insomnia component, trazodone 50mg at bedtime (acceptable during breastfeeding with monitoring for infant sedation). Zuranolone 50mg for 14 days is discussed as an option for rapid response given symptom severity. Close follow-up at 1 week is essential given the severity of presentation and the presence of intrusive thoughts.

18.5 Integration and Application

Perinatal prescribing requires a risk-benefit framework that accounts for two patients simultaneously. Preconception planning allows the safest medication transitions. During pregnancy, SSRIs are first-line for depression, lamotrigine is the preferred mood stabilizer, and antipsychotics should be continued when indicated for psychosis. Postpartum depression now has neurosteroid-based treatments (brexanolone and zuranolone) alongside established SSRIs. Lactation decisions are supported by regularly updated databases. Every prescribing decision should be documented with informed consent and coordinated with obstetric providers. The cross-reference to section 4.3 for pregnancy risk screening at every medication visit applies throughout reproductive-age prescribing.

Chapter 19.0: Pediatric Psychopharmacology

Prescribing psychiatric medications to children and adolescents carries responsibilities that adult prescribing does not. Developmental pharmacokinetics alter drug metabolism in ways that standard adult dosing cannot account for. FDA-approved indications are limited, forcing frequent off-label prescribing decisions. And the FDA black box warning on antidepressant suicidality in patients under 25 creates a monitoring obligation that must be documented at every visit.

19.1 Developmental Pharmacokinetics

Children are not small adults, and pediatric pharmacokinetics differ from adult pharmacokinetics in clinically meaningful ways. Hepatic metabolism is often faster in school-age children than in adults, meaning that weight-adjusted doses may be higher, not lower, than adult doses for some medications. Renal clearance is also increased relative to body size. By adolescence, metabolic rates approach adult levels (Stahl, 2021).

The practical implications: a 40 kg child on fluoxetine may require 20-40mg daily (the same absolute dose as an adult) because faster hepatic metabolism produces lower steady-state levels at a given milligram dose. Lithium clearance is higher in children, requiring more frequent dosing and closer level monitoring. Stimulant metabolism varies significantly with age, which is why formulation selection (duration of action matching the school day) matters as much as dose selection.

FDA-approved indications in pediatric psychiatry are limited. For depression, only fluoxetine (age 8+) and escitalopram (age 12+) have FDA approval. For anxiety, duloxetine has GAD approval for age 7+. For ADHD, multiple stimulant and non-stimulant options are approved (see section 11.2). For bipolar disorder, lithium (age 7+), aripiprazole, risperidone, quetiapine, olanzapine, and asenapine have various pediatric approvals. Off-label prescribing is common and appropriate when evidence supports it, but documentation of the rationale, informed consent from parents, and assent from the child are required (Walkup et al., 2008).

19.2 Pediatric Depression

The **black box warning** on antidepressants applies to all patients under 25 and requires specific monitoring: weekly visits for the first 4 weeks, biweekly for weeks 5-8, and at week 12. The warning reflects a small but statistically significant increase in suicidal ideation (not completed suicides) in pediatric antidepressant trials. The clinical reality is more nuanced: the risk of untreated depression (which carries a far higher suicide risk) generally outweighs the small risk of treatment-emergent suicidal ideation. But the monitoring requirement is non-negotiable and must be documented (Hammad et al., 2006).

Fluoxetine is the first-line antidepressant for pediatric depression based on the strongest evidence base. Starting dose: 10mg daily, titrating to 20mg after 1-2 weeks. The TADS study (Treatment for Adolescents with Depression Study) demonstrated that fluoxetine combined with CBT produced the best outcomes, with combination treatment achieving response rates of 71% compared to 61% for fluoxetine alone and 43% for CBT alone (March et al., 2004).

Escitalopram is second-line for ages 12 and above. Starting dose: 5mg, titrating to 10-20mg. Other SSRIs (sertraline, citalopram) are used off-label with reasonable supporting evidence.

When a patient fails two SSRI trials, augmentation follows the same principles as adult treatment (see section 5.3), with the caveat that metabolic monitoring for atypical antipsychotic augmentation is even more critical in developing youth. Weight gain during adolescence has long-term metabolic consequences that compound over decades.

TMS (transcranial magnetic stimulation) received FDA clearance for adolescent MDD (ages 15-21) in 2024, with multiple additional devices cleared in 2025. This represents a significant expansion of non-pharmacological treatment options for treatment-resistant adolescent depression (Stahl, 2021).

Consider the case of Jordan (composite example), a 15-year-old presenting with 4 months of depressed mood, social withdrawal, declining grades, sleep disruption, and passive suicidal ideation ("I sometimes wish I wouldn't wake up" without plan or intent). PHQ-A score is 16. Prior treatment: 8 weeks of school-based counseling without improvement. The treatment plan: fluoxetine 10mg daily, increasing to 20mg at week 2. Black box monitoring schedule documented: weekly visits for 4 weeks (phone check-ins if in-person visits are not feasible), biweekly for weeks 5-8. CBT referral placed. Parents educated on warning signs requiring immediate contact (new or worsening suicidal ideation, agitation, behavioral activation). Safety planning completed with the patient. The C-SSRS is administered at every visit and documented in the chart.

19.3 Pediatric Anxiety

The CAMS study (Child/Adolescent Anxiety Multimodal Study) demonstrated that **sertraline** combined with CBT produced the highest response rates (81%) for pediatric anxiety disorders, compared to 60% for sertraline alone and 55% for CBT alone (Walkup et al., 2008). SSRIs are first-line for pediatric anxiety. The "start low, go slow" principle applies: children with anxiety disorders are as sensitive to activation side effects as adults with panic disorder.

Duloxetine has FDA approval for GAD in children aged 7 and above, providing an SNRI option when SSRIs produce insufficient response. **Benzodiazepines** are generally avoided in pediatric populations due to paradoxical disinhibition risk, cognitive effects on developing brains, and dependence potential.

19.4 Pediatric Bipolar and Psychosis

Pediatric bipolar disorder diagnosis remains controversial, but when the diagnosis is established, pharmacotherapy follows adult principles with developmental modifications. Lithium is FDA-approved for ages 7 and above. Atypical antipsychotics (aripiprazole, risperidone, quetiapine, olanzapine) have pediatric bipolar approvals. Metabolic monitoring in youth is non-negotiable: the weight gain trajectory from early antipsychotic exposure predicts adult cardiometabolic risk (Correll et al., 2009).

First-episode psychosis in adolescents follows the FEP principles from section 10.1 with lower starting doses. Aripiprazole and risperidone are preferred first-line agents. Long-acting injectables are increasingly considered for adolescent patients with demonstrated adherence difficulties, though the evidence base is smaller than for adults.

19.5 Chapter Summary

Pediatric psychopharmacology requires developmental pharmacokinetic awareness, adherence to limited FDA-approved indications with documented off-label rationales, mandatory black box suicidality monitoring for antidepressants, and heightened metabolic vigilance for antipsychotics. Combination pharmacotherapy with evidence-based psychotherapy produces the best outcomes across depression and anxiety. The expansion of TMS to adolescents provides a new treatment modality for refractory cases.

Chapter 20.0: Geriatric Psychopharmacology

Prescribing for patients over 65 requires recalibrating everything you know about adult dosing. Hepatic metabolism slows. Renal clearance declines. Body composition shifts toward higher fat percentage, altering drug distribution. CNS sensitivity increases, meaning that the same blood level produces a stronger pharmacodynamic effect. The axiom "start low, go slow, but go" captures the clinical approach: conservative initiation, patient titration, but persistence toward therapeutic doses when tolerated. Undertreatment is as dangerous as overtreatment in geriatric psychiatry.

20.1 Pharmacologic Considerations

Age-related pharmacokinetic changes are predictable and systematic. Hepatic Phase I metabolism (CYP450 oxidation) declines with age while Phase II metabolism (conjugation, glucuronidation) is relatively preserved. This means medications primarily metabolized by CYP enzymes (most psychiatric medications) will reach higher steady-state levels in elderly patients at the same dose that younger adults receive. Renal clearance declines approximately 1% per year after age 40, making lithium and gabapentin dose adjustments essential. Decreased serum albumin reduces protein binding, increasing the free fraction of highly bound drugs like valproate and diazepam (Salzman, 2005).

The **Beers Criteria** (American Geriatrics Society, updated regularly) identify medications that are potentially inappropriate for older adults. Psychotropic entries include: all benzodiazepines (fall risk, cognitive impairment, delirium), first-generation antihistamines (anticholinergic burden), TCAs (anticholinergic effects, orthostasis, cardiac toxicity), and long-acting sulfonylureas. The prescriber should review the Beers list when initiating or inheriting any psychotropic regimen in an elderly patient (American Geriatrics Society, 2023).

Anticholinergic burden is a cumulative concept. Many psychiatric medications have anticholinergic properties: paroxetine, olanzapine, quetiapine, TCAs, hydroxyzine, diphenhydramine. In an elderly patient, these effects compound across medications and produce cognitive impairment, constipation (potentially progressing to ileus), urinary retention, blurred vision, and delirium. The Anticholinergic Cognitive Burden Scale quantifies this risk across a medication regimen. Reducing anticholinergic burden is often the single most impactful prescribing intervention in geriatric psychiatry (Stahl, 2021).

20.2 Geriatric Depression

SSRI selection in elderly patients should avoid paroxetine (the most anticholinergic SSRI with the highest drug interaction potential through CYP2D6 inhibition). **Sertraline** and **escitalopram** are preferred first-line agents. Citalopram is limited to 20mg daily in patients over 60 due to dose-dependent QTc prolongation (FDA guidance). **Venlafaxine** and **duloxetine** are reasonable SNRI options, with duloxetine offering the additional benefit of treating comorbid chronic pain (Stahl, 2021).

Mirtazapine is useful in elderly patients with depression accompanied by poor appetite, weight loss, and insomnia. The H1 antagonism produces appetite stimulation and sedation that may be therapeutic in the geriatric context. However, the sedation that is helpful at bedtime can persist as daytime grogginess, increasing fall risk.

Methylphenidate (5-20mg daily) has emerging evidence for apathetic depression in medically ill elderly patients, particularly those with advanced medical illness where faster onset than SSRIs is clinically important. It is used off-label and is generally well tolerated at low doses (Lavretsky et al., 2015).

ECT is highly effective in geriatric depression, with response rates exceeding 60-70%. It is particularly indicated for severe depression with psychotic features, active suicidality, food refusal, and treatment resistance. Cognitive side effects (primarily retrograde amnesia) require informed consent discussion, but ECT is generally safe in elderly patients without recent cerebrovascular events (Kellner et al., 2012).

Consider the case of Lorenzo (composite example), a 78-year-old man with new-onset depression following his wife's death 6 months ago. PHQ-9 is 20. He has lost 12 pounds, sleeps 3-4 hours nightly, reports feeling "empty" and hopeless, and has passive suicidal ideation. He takes metoprolol, amlodipine, and omeprazole. He lives alone. The prescribing assessment identifies multiple clinical targets: severe depression, significant weight loss, insomnia, and isolation. Mirtazapine 7.5mg at bedtime is initiated (targeting insomnia and appetite, starting at half the typical starting dose per geriatric protocol). Titration to 15mg at 2 weeks if tolerated. Omeprazole is a CYP2C19 inhibitor, but mirtazapine is primarily metabolized by CYP1A2 and CYP3A4, minimizing interaction concerns. Weekly phone check-ins for the first month given his isolation and suicidal ideation. Referral to bereavement support group. Follow-up PHQ-9 at 4 weeks to assess response trajectory.

20.3 Anxiety and Insomnia in Elderly

SSRIs and SNRIs are first-line for geriatric anxiety disorders, following the same selection principles as geriatric depression. **Buspirone** is safe in elderly patients without sedation or fall risk. **Benzodiazepines** should be avoided when possible in elderly patients: the Beers Criteria flag all benzodiazepines as potentially inappropriate due to increased sensitivity, prolonged half-lives (especially diazepam, which accumulates in adipose tissue), fall risk, cognitive impairment, and paradoxical agitation (American Geriatrics Society, 2023).

For insomnia, **suvorexant** (10mg, reduced from the standard 20mg starting dose) and **ramelteon** (8mg) are preferred because they avoid GABA-A agonism and its associated cognitive and fall risks. **Low-dose trazodone** (25-50mg) is widely used. **Z-drugs** should be avoided or used with extreme caution: the FDA recommends zolpidem 5mg (not 10mg) in elderly patients, and fall risk remains significant (Stahl, 2021).

20.4 Dementia Behavioral Management

The approach to behavioral and psychological symptoms of dementia (BPSD) is covered in section 15.2, but the geriatric prescribing context adds additional considerations.

The **2025 APA delirium guidelines** recommend against routine antipsychotic use for delirium prevention or treatment. Antipsychotics should be reserved for severe agitation or distress that threatens safety, and only after nonpharmacologic interventions and reversible contributors (pain, infection, constipation, medication effects, dehydration) have been addressed. For surgical patients, dexmedetomidine is suggested over other sedating agents for delirium prevention (APA, 2025).

When antipsychotics are used for BPSD, the black box warning for increased mortality in elderly patients with dementia-related psychosis applies to all antipsychotics. **Brexpiprazole** is the only agent with specific FDA approval for agitation in Alzheimer's dementia (see section 15.2). All antipsychotic use in dementia should be time-limited with regular reassessment of continued need.

20.5 Deprescribing Strategies

Systematic medication review in elderly patients frequently identifies psychotropic medications that were started years ago for indications that no longer exist, at doses that are no longer appropriate, or in combinations that produce cumulative toxicity. Deprescribing is an active clinical skill, not passive neglect.

Benzodiazepine tapering in long-term elderly users follows the 2025 guidelines (section 7.4), with the additional consideration that elderly patients may be more sensitive to withdrawal symptoms and require even slower tapers (2.5-5% reduction every 2-4 weeks). **Anticholinergic reduction** involves identifying all medications contributing to anticholinergic burden and systematically replacing or eliminating them. **Antipsychotic reassessment** in dementia patients should occur every 3-6 months, with dose reduction trials when behavioral symptoms have been stable (Stahl, 2021).

Consider the case of Dorothy (identifying details changed), an 82-year-old woman with mild Alzheimer's dementia admitted to her daughter's home after a fall. Her medication list includes: lorazepam 0.5mg twice daily (prescribed 8 years ago for "anxiety"), quetiapine 100mg at bedtime (started 3 years ago for "agitation" at a previous facility), diphenhydramine 25mg nightly (self-administered for sleep), mirtazapine 15mg at bedtime (for depression), donepezil 10mg daily, and lisinopril 10mg. The geriatric prescribing assessment identifies three high-risk medications: lorazepam (Beers Criteria, fall risk, cognitive impairment), diphenhydramine (anticholinergic burden, delirium risk, Beers Criteria), and quetiapine (black box dementia warning, metabolic effects, sedation compounding fall risk). The deprescribing plan: (1) Discontinue diphenhydramine immediately (no taper needed). (2) Begin lorazepam taper per 2025 guidelines, reducing by 0.125mg every 2-3 weeks. (3) Reassess quetiapine indication: if "agitation" is no longer present or was never clearly documented, begin gradual dose reduction with behavioral monitoring. (4) Maintain mirtazapine (targeting depression, insomnia, and appetite). (5) Continue donepezil. The result: reduced fall risk, reduced anticholinergic burden, and a medication regimen aligned with current evidence.

20.6 Concluding Thoughts

Geriatric psychopharmacology demands slower titration, lower target doses, systematic anticholinergic burden assessment, Beers Criteria awareness, and proactive deprescribing. The 2025 delirium guidelines restrict antipsychotic use in delirium management. Benzodiazepine avoidance or tapering is a clinical priority. Undertreatment of depression is as problematic as overtreatment with inappropriate agents.

Chapter 21.0: Medical Comorbidity Prescribing

Your patients do not arrive with isolated psychiatric diagnoses. They arrive with diabetes, chronic kidney disease, heart failure, hepatic cirrhosis, chronic pain, seizure disorders, and thyroid dysfunction. Every one of these medical conditions changes the prescribing calculus for psychiatric medications. Some changes are pharmacokinetic (the body processes the medication differently). Others are pharmacodynamic (the medication's effects interact with the medical condition). And some are simply additive risk (the side effect profile of the psychiatric medication worsens the medical condition). This chapter provides the clinical decision framework for each of these intersections.

21.1 Hepatic Impairment

The liver metabolizes the majority of psychiatric medications, making hepatic impairment one of the most consequential medical comorbidities for the prescriber. Reduced hepatic function means slower drug metabolism, higher steady-state drug levels, and increased side effect risk at standard doses.

Medications requiring dose reduction: Most psychotropic agents metabolized by CYP450 enzymes require dose reduction in moderate-to-severe hepatic impairment. General guidance is a 50% starting dose reduction, with slower titration and closer monitoring. **Preferred agents** in hepatic impairment include **paliperidone** (primarily renally eliminated, minimal hepatic metabolism), **escitalopram** (relatively low hepatic burden), and **gabapentin/pregabalin** (renally eliminated). **Medications to avoid** in severe hepatic disease: valproate (hepatotoxic, contraindicated), nefazodone (black box warning for hepatic failure), duloxetine (contraindicated in substantial alcohol use or chronic liver disease), and high-dose acetaminophen combinations (Stahl, 2021).

Consider the case of Miguel (composite example), a 58-year-old man with alcohol-related cirrhosis (Child-Pugh Class B) and comorbid major depression. He has been sober for 14 months and is maintained on naltrexone for AUD (section 13.1). His depression was previously managed with duloxetine 60mg, but his hepatologist flagged the duloxetine as contraindicated given his hepatic status. The prescriber transitions to escitalopram 5mg (starting at half the typical dose, with titration to 10mg after 2 weeks based on tolerability). Naltrexone is continued with LFT monitoring every 3 months. Paliperidone would be an option if antipsychotic treatment were needed, given its renal elimination pathway.

21.2 Renal Impairment

Lithium is the psychiatric medication most affected by renal impairment because it is eliminated entirely by the kidneys. In patients with decreased GFR, lithium clearance drops proportionally, requiring dose reduction (often 25-50% of standard dosing) and more frequent level monitoring. As renal function declines, some providers transition to alternative mood stabilizers. Chronic lithium use itself can cause nephrogenic diabetes insipidus and, over decades, interstitial nephritis. Renal function (creatinine, GFR) should be monitored every 6 months in all lithium patients (Malhi et al., 2017).

Gabapentin and pregabalin are renally eliminated and require dose adjustment based on creatinine clearance. At GFR below 30 mL/min, gabapentin maximum dose drops to 300mg daily. **Paliperidone** requires dose reduction in renal impairment (unlike its parent compound risperidone, which is primarily hepatically metabolized). **Desvenlafaxine** requires dose reduction to 50mg daily (or every other day) in severe renal impairment. Most other psychiatric medications do not require renal dose adjustment but deserve monitoring in the context of polypharmacy and fluctuating renal function (Stahl, 2021).

21.3 Cardiovascular Considerations

QTc prolongation is the primary cardiac risk in psychiatric prescribing. Medications with the highest QTc risk include ziprasidone, thioridazine, IV haloperidol, citalopram (dose-dependent, capped at 40mg in general and 20mg in elderly), and certain drug combinations (see section 2.3 for the QTc interaction table). Baseline ECG is indicated before starting these agents and when risk factors are present (personal or family history of cardiac arrhythmia, electrolyte abnormalities, concurrent QTc-prolonging medications, structural heart disease). A QTc above 500ms or an increase of more than 60ms from baseline is a threshold for immediate medication reassessment (Beach et al., 2013).

Post-myocardial infarction depression affects 15-20% of MI patients and doubles mortality risk when untreated. SSRIs are the preferred treatment: the SADHART trial demonstrated that sertraline is safe and effective in post-ACS depression without increasing cardiac events. TCAs are contraindicated post-MI due to cardiac conduction effects and arrhythmia risk (Glassman et al., 2002).

Venlafaxine produces dose-dependent blood pressure elevation, particularly above 225mg daily. Monitor blood pressure at baseline, after each dose increase, and at regular intervals during maintenance. Patients with uncontrolled hypertension may require an alternative antidepressant.

21.4 Metabolic Syndrome

The metabolic risk hierarchy of atypical antipsychotics is discussed in section 10.2. When an antipsychotic is required in a patient with existing diabetes or metabolic syndrome, **weight-neutral options** include aripiprazole, cariprazine, ziprasidone, lurasidone, and brexpiprazole. **Cobenfy** (xanomeline/trospium), with its non-dopaminergic mechanism, demonstrates a favorable metabolic profile and may be particularly appropriate for patients with significant metabolic risk who require antipsychotic treatment (Kaul et al., 2024).

Metformin (500-2000mg daily) has evidence for attenuating antipsychotic-induced weight gain when initiated within the first few months of antipsychotic treatment. Starting metformin concurrently with a high-metabolic-risk antipsychotic (olanzapine, clozapine, quetiapine) is increasingly considered a proactive prescribing strategy rather than a reactive one (Stahl, 2021).

21.5 Chronic Pain Integration

The intersection of chronic pain and psychiatric illness creates prescribing opportunities when a single medication can address both conditions.

Duloxetine (60-120mg) has FDA approval for MDD, GAD, diabetic peripheral neuropathy, fibromyalgia, and chronic musculoskeletal pain. It is the single most efficient medication choice when depression and chronic pain co-occur. **Gabapentin** (300-3600mg) and **pregabalin** (150-600mg) address anxiety and neuropathic pain simultaneously. **TCAs** at sub-antidepressant doses (amitriptyline 10-50mg, nortriptyline 10-50mg at bedtime) are effective for neuropathic pain and fibromyalgia, though anticholinergic effects limit their use in elderly patients (Stahl, 2021).

Cyclobenzaprine sublingual (Tonmya), approved in 2025 for fibromyalgia, uses a low-dose sublingual formulation that targets the sleep-pain cycle. It acts on serotonergic and noradrenergic pathways at doses below the muscle relaxant threshold, reducing central pain sensitization and improving sleep architecture.

The critical prescribing caution: avoid combining opioids with benzodiazepines. This combination carries a black box warning for respiratory depression and death. When patients present on both, a tapering plan for one or both agents should be prioritized (section 7.4 for benzodiazepine tapering).

Consider the case of Tanisha (identifying details changed), a 47-year-old woman with fibromyalgia, MDD (PHQ-9: 17), and GAD (GAD-7: 14). She takes tramadol 50mg three times daily for pain and lorazepam 0.5mg twice daily for anxiety. Both were prescribed by her primary care provider. The psychiatric prescribing plan addresses all three conditions while reducing polypharmacy risk: (1) Initiate duloxetine 30mg for 1 week, then increase to 60mg (targeting depression, anxiety, and fibromyalgia pain simultaneously). (2) Discontinue tramadol when duloxetine reaches 60mg (serotonin syndrome risk with the combination, and duloxetine addresses the pain indication). (3) Begin lorazepam taper per 2025 guidelines once duloxetine reaches therapeutic effect (typically 4-6 weeks). (4) Add gabapentin 300mg at bedtime for residual pain and sleep support if needed. (5) Discuss Tonmya as an option if the sleep-pain cycle remains inadequately addressed. The net result: three conditions treated with one or two medications instead of multiple agents with overlapping risks.

21.6 Seizure and Thyroid Disorders

Seizure threshold lowering is a pharmacodynamic concern with several psychiatric medications. **Bupropion** lowers seizure threshold, with risk increasing above 450mg daily and in patients with predisposing conditions (eating disorders, alcohol withdrawal, history of seizures). **Clozapine** is associated with dose-dependent seizure risk (approximately 5% at doses above 600mg). **Chlorpromazine** lowers seizure threshold more than other antipsychotics. When prescribing for patients with epilepsy, favor medications with no or minimal seizure threshold effects (SSRIs, SNRIs other than bupropion, most atypical antipsychotics) and monitor closely when seizure-lowering agents are unavoidable.

Mood stabilizers with anticonvulsant properties (valproate, carbamazepine, lamotrigine) offer a dual benefit in patients with comorbid epilepsy and bipolar disorder. Drug interactions with antiepileptic medications require careful CYP450 review (section 2.2), particularly carbamazepine's pan-induction effects.

Lithium-induced hypothyroidism occurs in 5-35% of patients on long-term lithium therapy. TSH monitoring every 6 months is standard practice. Treatment with levothyroxine is straightforward and does not require lithium discontinuation. **T3 (triiodothyronine) augmentation** at 25-50mcg daily for depression (section 5.3) requires monitoring to distinguish augmentation effects from treatment of subclinical hypothyroidism (Malhi et al., 2017).

21.7 Summary and Recommendations

Medical comorbidity prescribing requires systematic assessment of how each medical condition alters the pharmacokinetics, pharmacodynamics, and side effect risk of psychiatric medications. Hepatic impairment demands dose reduction for CYP-metabolized drugs. Renal impairment affects lithium, gabapentin, pregabalin, and paliperidone. Cardiac risk centers on QTc monitoring. Metabolic syndrome should drive antipsychotic selection toward weight-neutral agents. Chronic pain presents opportunities for dual-purpose medications. Seizure and thyroid disorders interact with specific psychiatric medications in predictable, manageable ways. The cross-references throughout this chapter connect to the specific disease-based prescribing chapters where these comorbidity adjustments are embedded in the decision trees.

Chapter 22.0: Psychiatric Emergencies

Psychiatric emergencies demand rapid pharmacological decisions under pressure. The prescriber who has rehearsed these scenarios mentally is the prescriber who acts decisively when a patient is acutely agitated, develops serotonin syndrome, or presents with neuroleptic malignant syndrome. This chapter provides the recognition criteria and treatment protocols for the emergencies you are most likely to encounter.

22.1 Acute Agitation Management

Verbal de-escalation is always the first intervention. When pharmacological management is necessary, the goal is rapid sedation sufficient to ensure safety without excessive sedation that compromises airway protection or prevents ongoing assessment.

Oral options (preferred when the patient will accept oral medication): Lorazepam 1-2mg, olanzapine ODT 5-10mg (orally disintegrating tablet placed on the tongue), risperidone liquid 1-2mg, or haloperidol 2-5mg with diphenhydramine 25-50mg (to prevent dystonia).

IM options (when oral administration is refused or impractical): The classic combination is **haloperidol 5mg + lorazepam 2mg + diphenhydramine 50mg IM**, which provides antipsychotic, anxiolytic, and EPS-prophylactic coverage simultaneously. **Olanzapine 10mg IM** is effective and rapid-onset. **Ziprasidone 10-20mg IM** is an alternative when metabolic concerns exist.

Critical safety point: Never combine IM olanzapine with IM benzodiazepines. This combination carries a risk of respiratory depression, hypotension, and death. If a patient has received IM olanzapine, wait at least one hour before administering a benzodiazepine, and vice versa. This is a non-negotiable prescribing rule (Wilson et al., 2012).

For agitation in the context of known or suspected substance intoxication: benzodiazepines are preferred over antipsychotics for stimulant intoxication (cocaine, methamphetamine) because antipsychotics may lower the seizure threshold and worsen hyperthermia. For alcohol intoxication-related agitation, haloperidol is preferred because benzodiazepines compound CNS depression (Stahl, 2021).

22.2 Serotonin Syndrome

Recognition: The Hunter Criteria provide the most clinically useful diagnostic framework. In the presence of a serotonergic agent, serotonin syndrome is diagnosed if any of the following are present: spontaneous clonus, inducible clonus with agitation or diaphoresis, ocular clonus with agitation or diaphoresis, tremor with hyperreflexia, or hypertonia with temperature above 38 degrees Celsius (Boyer & Shannon, 2005).

The clinical triad is: (1) **Autonomic instability** (hyperthermia, tachycardia, hypertension, diaphoresis, mydriasis). (2) **Neuromuscular hyperactivity** (clonus, hyperreflexia, myoclonus, tremor, rigidity). (3) **Altered mental status** (agitation, confusion, delirium).

Causative combinations most commonly involve: SSRI/SNRI + MAOI (the highest-risk combination), SSRI + tramadol, SSRI + triptans (lower risk), SSRI + linezolid, SSRI + methylene blue, and high-dose SSRI/SNRI monotherapy (rare). The prescriber's role is prevention through awareness of these combinations (section 2.3).

Management: (1) Discontinue all serotonergic agents immediately. (2) **Cyproheptadine** 12mg initial dose (crushed via NG tube if patient cannot swallow), followed by 2mg every 2 hours as needed for symptom control. (3) Benzodiazepines for agitation and myoclonus. (4) External cooling for hyperthermia (avoid antipyretics, which are ineffective because the hyperthermia is caused by muscular hyperactivity, not hypothalamic set-point elevation). (5) Intubation and paralysis with nondepolarizing agents for severe cases with temperature above 41 degrees Celsius (Boyer & Shannon, 2005).

Most cases resolve within 24-72 hours after discontinuation of the offending agents. Mild cases (tremor, hyperreflexia, mild agitation) may require only observation and discontinuation.

22.3 Neuroleptic Malignant Syndrome

Recognition: NMS presents with the tetrad of (1) **fever** (often above 40 degrees Celsius), (2) **lead-pipe rigidity** (generalized, not clonus as in serotonin syndrome), (3) **autonomic instability** (tachycardia, labile blood pressure, diaphoresis), and (4) **altered consciousness** (confusion progressing to stupor or coma). Laboratory findings include markedly elevated CK (often above 1000 U/L, sometimes above 10,000), leukocytosis, elevated LFTs, and metabolic acidosis (Strawn et al., 2007).

NMS develops in response to dopamine antagonists (antipsychotics most commonly) or rapid withdrawal of dopaminergic agents (levodopa, amantadine). It can occur at any point during treatment, even after stable dosing for months or years, though it most commonly appears within the first 2 weeks of a new antipsychotic or dose increase.

Management: (1) Stop the offending antipsychotic immediately. (2) **Dantrolene** 1-2.5 mg/kg IV for muscle rigidity and hyperthermia (acts directly on skeletal muscle to reduce contraction). (3) **Bromocriptine** 2.5mg orally every 8 hours (dopamine agonist that counteracts the D2 blockade causing NMS). (4) Aggressive IV fluids for renal protection (rhabdomyolysis from CK elevation can cause acute kidney injury). (5) External cooling. (6) ICU monitoring. Mortality rates range from 5-20% with treatment (Strawn et al., 2007).

Re-challenge considerations: After NMS resolution (typically 1-2 weeks), if antipsychotic treatment is still indicated, wait at least 2 weeks. Choose a structurally different antipsychotic with lower D2 binding potency (e.g., if NMS occurred on haloperidol, consider quetiapine or clozapine). Start at the lowest possible dose and titrate very slowly.

Consider the case of David (composite example), a 24-year-old male with schizophrenia who was started on haloperidol 10mg IM in the emergency department for acute psychosis 3 days ago. He now presents with temperature of 40.2 degrees Celsius, diffuse muscle rigidity, tachycardia (heart rate 128), and altered consciousness (confused, responds only to loud verbal stimuli). CK is 8,400 U/L. WBC is 14,200. The recognition is immediate: this is NMS until proven otherwise. Management: haloperidol is discontinued. Dantrolene IV is started. Bromocriptine 2.5mg is administered via NG tube. Aggressive IV normal saline is initiated for renal protection. Transfer to ICU for continuous monitoring. Urine output is tracked hourly as an indicator of renal function. The clinical lesson: NMS can develop rapidly, even with a single high-dose antipsychotic injection. Vigilance during the first 2 weeks of any new antipsychotic is essential.

22.4 Lithium Toxicity

Mild toxicity (1.5-2.0 mEq/L): Nausea, vomiting, diarrhea, coarse tremor, drowsiness. Management: hold lithium, IV normal saline for hydration, serial lithium levels every 6 hours, identify precipitating cause (dehydration, new NSAID, ACE inhibitor, thiazide diuretic).

Moderate toxicity (2.0-2.5 mEq/L): Ataxia, slurred speech, confusion, fasciculations, increased deep tendon reflexes. Management: as above with more aggressive IV hydration. Consider whole bowel irrigation if recent large ingestion.

Severe toxicity (above 2.5 mEq/L): Seizures, renal failure, coma, cardiovascular collapse. Management: **hemodialysis** is indicated for levels above 4.0 mEq/L, levels above 2.5 with renal impairment, or any level with severe neurological symptoms. Rebound lithium elevation is common after dialysis as lithium redistributes from tissue compartments; repeat levels 6-8 hours post-dialysis (Decker et al., 2015).

Prevention is the prescriber's primary role. Lithium drug interactions (section 2.3), hydration counseling, and level monitoring protocols (section 4.2) prevent the vast majority of toxicity episodes.

22.5 Psychotropic Overdose

TCA overdose is a medical emergency. Cardiotoxicity (QRS widening, arrhythmias, hypotension), seizures, and anticholinergic delirium constitute the lethal triad. Management: **sodium bicarbonate** (1-2 mEq/kg IV bolus, targeting serum pH of 7.45-7.55) is the primary treatment for cardiac conduction abnormalities. Activated charcoal within 1-2 hours of ingestion. Benzodiazepines for seizures (avoid phenytoin, which worsens cardiac conduction). Monitor QRS interval continuously: QRS above 100ms predicts seizure risk, above 160ms predicts arrhythmia risk (Woolf et al., 2007).

SSRI/SNRI overdose is generally less lethal than TCA overdose. Serotonin syndrome symptoms may develop (see section 22.2). Citalopram and escitalopram carry QTc prolongation risk in overdose, requiring ECG monitoring. Venlafaxine overdose carries seizure risk and possible cardiac effects at very high doses.

Antipsychotic overdose produces sedation, hypotension, anticholinergic effects (with older agents), and QTc prolongation. Quetiapine overdose is increasingly common and can produce significant sedation, tachycardia, and hypotension. Management is primarily supportive with airway protection and hemodynamic support.

Prescribing for safety: When prescribing to patients at suicide risk, consider lethality in overdose. Avoid TCAs, prefer SSRIs. Limit quantities dispensed (2-week supplies for high-risk patients). Document the risk assessment and prescribing rationale per the framework in section 4.3.

22.6 Suicidal Crisis Pharmacology

Medication plays a supporting role in suicidal crises alongside safety planning, means restriction, increased monitoring, and often hospitalization. Specific pharmacological considerations:

Lithium has the strongest evidence for suicide reduction in mood disorders. A meta-analysis of 48 randomized trials found that lithium significantly reduced suicide deaths, deliberate self-harm, and all-cause mortality in patients with mood disorders (Cipriani et al., 2013). This anti-suicidal effect appears independent of lithium's mood-stabilizing properties.

Clozapine is the only antipsychotic with specific FDA indication for reducing suicidal behavior in schizophrenia and schizoaffective disorder, based on the InterSePT trial demonstrating 26% reduction in suicidal behavior versus olanzapine (Meltzer et al., 2003).

Esketamine REMS requirements include observation for suicidal ideation and behavior during and after administration. While the speed of esketamine's antidepressant effect is relevant in suicidal patients with TRD, it is not approved as an anti-suicidal agent per se.

Means restriction counseling is a prescribing-adjacent intervention: when a patient in crisis has access to firearms, lethal medications, or other means, the prescriber should counsel on temporary means restriction and document this conversation. Limiting prescribed quantities and avoiding lethal-in-overdose agents

(TCAs, lithium in impulsive patients without monitoring support) are direct prescribing decisions that affect suicide risk.

22.7 Essential Points

Psychiatric emergencies require rapid recognition and protocol-based treatment. Acute agitation management follows a hierarchy: verbal de-escalation, oral medication, IM medication (never combine IM olanzapine with IM benzodiazepines). Serotonin syndrome is treated with agent discontinuation, cyproheptadine, and supportive care. NMS is treated with antipsychotic discontinuation, dantrolene, and bromocriptine. Lithium toxicity management escalates from hydration through hemodialysis based on level and symptoms. TCA overdose requires sodium bicarbonate. Suicide risk pharmacology includes lithium for mood disorders and clozapine for schizophrenia spectrum disorders. Prevention through safe prescribing practices (interaction awareness, means restriction counseling, limited quantities for high-risk patients) is the most effective emergency intervention.

Part IV: Practical Tools and References

Chapters 23 through 26: Algorithms, Interaction Tables, Monitoring, Patient Education

Chapter 23.0: Prescribing Decision Algorithms

Every prescribing decision follows a logic. The decision trees in this chapter make that logic explicit. They are not substitutes for clinical judgment. They are frameworks that ensure you ask the right questions in the right order, consider the evidence-based options at each branch point, and document a rational prescribing pathway that another clinician could follow and understand.

These algorithms distill the diagnosis-based prescribing guidance from Chapters 5.0 through 17.0 into visual decision pathways. Use them as rapid-access tools during clinical encounters. When the algorithm points you toward a specific medication or strategy, the corresponding chapter provides the detailed dosing, monitoring, and clinical nuance behind that recommendation.

23.1 Depressed Mood Algorithm

The master algorithm for a patient presenting with depressed mood begins with diagnostic clarification, not medication selection.

Step 1: Confirm the diagnosis. Administer the PHQ-9 (section 4.1). Score of 10 or above warrants pharmacotherapy consideration. Administer the MDQ to screen for bipolar features. If the MDQ is positive, proceed to section 6.1 for bipolar evaluation before prescribing an antidepressant. Rule out medical contributors: obtain baseline TSH, CBC, and metabolic panel. Review the medication list for depressogenic agents (corticosteroids, interferon, beta-blockers, hormonal contraceptives). Assess substance use with AUDIT-C. If active substance use is identified, address concurrently per section 13.4.

Step 2: Identify the dominant symptom cluster. This determines first-line medication selection. Sadness and anxiety predominant: SSRI (sertraline 50mg or escitalopram 10mg). Fatigue and psychomotor retardation predominant: SNRI (duloxetine 60mg or venlafaxine XR 75mg) or bupropion (150mg XL). Insomnia and appetite loss predominant: mirtazapine (15mg at bedtime). Comorbid chronic pain: duloxetine (60mg). Sexual dysfunction as a primary concern: bupropion (150-300mg XL). These are starting points, not rigid prescriptions. The prescriber adjusts based on drug interactions (section 2.2), pharmacogenomic data if available (section 3.2), medical comorbidities (Chapter 21.0), and patient preference.

Step 3: Assess response at defined intervals. At 2 weeks: any improvement? If none and side effects are intolerable, consider switching. If none but tolerable, optimize dose. At 4 weeks: has the PHQ-9 decreased by at least 25%? If yes, continue and optimize. If no, reassess adherence, dose adequacy, and diagnosis. At 6-8 weeks at therapeutic dose: has the PHQ-9 decreased by 50% or more (response)? Is the PHQ-9 below 5 (remission)?

Step 4: Manage partial response. If the patient has achieved 25-49% reduction after an adequate trial, augmentation is preferred over switching. First-line augmentation: aripiprazole (2-5mg, titrate to effect), brexpiprazole (0.5-1mg), or lithium (300-600mg, targeting level 0.4-0.8 mEq/L). Alternative augmentation: buspirone (15-30mg divided), T3 (25-50mcg), lumateperone (42mg). If augmentation fails, switch to a different class.

Step 5: Treatment-resistant pathway. After failure of two adequate trials of different medication classes: rule out pseudo-resistance (adherence, diagnosis, comorbidities, pharmacokinetics). Consider pharmacogenomic testing (section 3.1). Options: esketamine monotherapy (clinic-based), Auvelity (dextromethorphan/bupropion), MAOI (tranylcypromine, phenelzine, or transdermal selegiline), or TCA trial with therapeutic drug monitoring. For severe, life-threatening TRD: ECT referral. See section 5.4 for detailed TRD management.

Consider the case of Amina (composite example), a 36-year-old woman presenting with PHQ-9 of 18, dominant symptoms of fatigue, poor concentration, and chronic lower back pain, with no prior psychiatric treatment. Following the algorithm: Step 1 confirms MDD (MDQ negative, TSH normal, no substance use). Step 2 identifies fatigue and pain as dominant, pointing to duloxetine 60mg. Step 3 at 4 weeks shows PHQ-9 of 12 (33% reduction, partial response at sub-optimal dose). Duloxetine is increased to 90mg. At 8 weeks, PHQ-9 is 8 (56% reduction, response but not remission). She continues at 90mg with reassessment at 12 weeks. The algorithm provided the structure. Clinical judgment refined each decision.

23.2 Anxiety Presentation Algorithm

Step 1: Differentiate the anxiety subtype. GAD presents with persistent, excessive worry across multiple domains lasting 6+ months. Panic disorder presents with recurrent unexpected panic attacks with anticipatory anxiety. Social anxiety presents as marked fear of social or performance situations. PTSD presents with re-experiencing, avoidance, hyperarousal, and negative cognitions following a traumatic event (proceed to section 9.1 for the PTSD-specific algorithm). OCD presents with obsessions and/or compulsions (proceed to section 8.1 for the OCD-specific algorithm).

Step 2: First-line pharmacotherapy by subtype. GAD: SSRI or SNRI at standard doses (sertraline 50-200mg, escitalopram 10-20mg, duloxetine 60-120mg, venlafaxine XR 75-225mg). Panic disorder: SSRI at half the usual starting dose (sertraline 25mg, escitalopram 5mg), titrating slowly. Social anxiety (generalized): SSRI or SNRI at higher-end doses. Social anxiety (performance only): propranolol 10-40mg PRN 30-60 minutes before performance.

Step 3: Benzodiazepine decision. Is a short-term bridge needed while waiting for SSRI/SNRI onset? If yes: clonazepam 0.25-0.5mg twice daily or lorazepam 0.5-1mg twice daily for a maximum of 4 weeks, with taper plan established before the first prescription. If the patient has a history of substance use disorder: do not prescribe benzodiazepines. Use hydroxyzine (25-50mg as needed) or gabapentin (300mg as needed) as alternatives for acute symptom relief during the SSRI onset period.

Step 4: Partial response management. After 6-8 weeks at adequate SSRI/SNRI dose: augment with buspirone (15-60mg daily), gabapentin (300-1800mg daily), or pregabalin (150-600mg daily). If SSRIs and SNRIs have both failed: consider mirtazapine (15-45mg), TCA (clomipramine for panic/social anxiety), or referral for specialized anxiety treatment.

Step 5: Benzodiazepine tapering for chronic users. Follow the 2025 Joint Clinical Practice Guideline (section 7.4): 5-10% dose reduction every 2-4 weeks, hyperbolic tapering at lower doses, adjunctive CBT-I and behavioral supports, and conversion to longer-acting equivalents when appropriate.

23.3 Psychosis Presentation Algorithm

Step 1: Distinguish first-episode psychosis from chronic schizophrenia from substance-induced psychosis. Urine drug screen is mandatory. If positive for stimulants, cannabis, or hallucinogens, observe for 48-72 hours off substances before diagnosing a primary psychotic disorder. If the patient has a known schizophrenia diagnosis, proceed to Step 3.

Step 2: First-episode psychosis. Select an atypical antipsychotic based on the metabolic risk profile (section 10.2). Preferred agents: aripiprazole (10-15mg), risperidone (1-3mg). Start at approximately half the chronic schizophrenia dose. Plan for 1-2 years of treatment following first-episode remission, with gradual dose reduction considered thereafter.

Step 3: Chronic schizophrenia. Optimize current antipsychotic dose if response is partial. If the patient has failed the current agent at adequate dose for 6-8 weeks, switch to a different antipsychotic class. Consider Cobenfy (xanomeline/trospium 125mg/30mg twice daily) for patients with metabolic contraindications to dopamine-blocking agents.

Step 4: Treatment-resistant schizophrenia. After failure of two adequate antipsychotic trials of different classes: clozapine. See section 10.3 for titration, monitoring (post-2025 REMS elimination), and management protocols. Clozapine is the only evidence-based treatment for TRS, and delay in initiating it when criteria are met constitutes suboptimal care.

Step 5: Side effect management pathway. TD develops: initiate valbenazine (40-80mg) or deutetrabenazine (12-48mg) per section 10.4. Significant weight gain: switch to lower-metabolic-risk agent or add metformin. Akathisia: reduce dose, switch agent, add propranolol (20-80mg). Hyperprolactinemia: switch to aripiprazole or cariprazine. QTc prolongation: obtain ECG, reduce dose or switch agent, correct electrolytes.

Consider the case of Rafael (composite example), a 22-year-old male presenting with 6 months of auditory hallucinations, paranoid ideation, and functional decline. Urine drug screen is negative. BMI is 22, fasting glucose is 88, and lipid panel is normal. This is first-episode psychosis with a favorable metabolic baseline. Following the algorithm: aripiprazole is initiated at 10mg daily, with a plan to titrate to 15mg at week 2 if tolerated. Metabolic monitoring is scheduled per section 4.2. He is referred for coordinated specialty care (CSC), which integrates medication management, psychotherapy, supported education/employment, and family education. At 4 weeks, PANSS positive symptom score has decreased by 40%. Aripiprazole is maintained at 15mg. The algorithm structured the approach. Coordinated specialty care provides the full-spectrum treatment envelope.

23.4 Mood Instability Algorithm

Step 1: Confirm bipolar spectrum diagnosis. Administer the MDQ. Review history for discrete manic or hypomanic episodes (elevated mood, decreased need for sleep, grandiosity, increased goal-directed activity, impulsivity lasting at least 4 days for hypomania or 7 days for mania). Distinguish bipolar I (mania) from bipolar II (hypomania with major depression) from cyclothymia (chronic sub-threshold mood fluctuations).

Step 2: Determine current episode polarity. Acute mania: proceed to lithium, valproate, or atypical antipsychotic per section 6.2. Acute bipolar depression: proceed to quetiapine, lurasidone, cariprazine, lumateperone, or lamotrigine per section 6.3. Mixed features: avoid antidepressants, prioritize atypical antipsychotics and mood stabilizers. Euthymic (maintenance): proceed to long-term mood stabilizer selection per section 6.4.

Step 3: Special considerations. Rapid cycling (4+ episodes per year): optimize mood stabilizers, minimize antidepressants, check thyroid function, address substance use. Reproductive-age patient: avoid valproate (section 18.1), prefer lamotrigine, discuss contraception. Suicidal risk: lithium's anti-suicidal properties make it a priority consideration (section 22.6).

23.5 Additional Quick Algorithms

Insomnia: CBT-I referral first. If medication needed: sleep onset difficulty, use ramelteon 8mg or suvorexant 10mg. Sleep maintenance difficulty: low-dose doxepin 3-6mg or lemborexant 5mg. Short-term only (2-4 weeks): zolpidem 5mg (elderly) or 10mg (adults under 65). Chronic benzodiazepine/Z-drug use: taper per section 7.4. See section 12.1 for full insomnia management.

ADHD: Screen for comorbidities first (section 11.1). Uncomplicated ADHD: stimulant (lisdexamfetamine 30mg or methylphenidate ER 18mg), titrate to response. If first stimulant class fails, try the other class. If stimulants contraindicated or ineffective: atomoxetine, viloxazine ER, or guanfacine ER. Complex ADHD: stabilize comorbid condition first (mood, anxiety, SUD), then address ADHD. See section 11.4 for complex presentations.

PTSD: Sleep disturbance first (prazosin 1mg, titrate to effect). Then daytime symptoms (sertraline 50-200mg or venlafaxine XR 75-225mg). Taper benzodiazepines if present. Augment with atypical antipsychotic if partial SSRI response. See section 9.1 for the full PTSD algorithm.

Substance use disorder: AUD: naltrexone (oral 50mg daily or Vivitrol 380mg monthly) or acamprosate (666mg TID). OUD: buprenorphine/naloxone induction (traditional or micro-dosing), maintenance 16-24mg, consider Sublocade transition. Tobacco: varenicline (0.5mg daily for 3 days, 0.5mg BID for 4 days, then 1mg BID) or bupropion SR (150mg BID). See Chapter 13.0 for full SUD management.

23.6 Using the Algorithms Clinically

These algorithms are designed for two clinical contexts. The first is the real-time prescribing encounter: you have a patient in front of you, a presenting complaint, and 15 minutes to make a decision. The algorithm gets you to the decision point. The referenced section provides the clinical detail. The second context is case review and supervision: when you are reviewing a prescribing decision with a colleague, trainee, or supervising physician, the algorithm provides a shared framework for discussing the clinical logic.

The algorithms do not capture every clinical nuance. A patient's preference, insurance formulary restrictions, prior treatment history, and psychosocial context all modify the algorithmic recommendation. The algorithm tells you what the evidence supports. You tell the algorithm what this specific patient needs.

23.7 Key Takeaways

Decision algorithms provide structured, evidence-based pathways from clinical presentation to medication selection. The depression algorithm moves from diagnostic confirmation through symptom-matched first-line selection, defined response benchmarks, augmentation strategies, and treatment-resistant pathways. The anxiety algorithm differentiates subtypes, applies subtype-specific pharmacotherapy, and incorporates benzodiazepine management. The psychosis algorithm distinguishes first-episode from chronic from substance-induced presentations and includes the treatment-resistant pathway to clozapine. The mood instability algorithm addresses episode polarity and special considerations. Quick algorithms for insomnia, ADHD, PTSD, and SUDs provide rapid-access prescribing frameworks. All algorithms cross-reference the detailed clinical content in their corresponding chapters.

Chapter 24.0: Drug Interaction Reference

Drug interactions kill patients. That statement is not hyperbole. Serotonin syndrome from an SSRI combined with tramadol, torsades de pointes from accumulating QTc-prolonging agents, lithium toxicity from a newly prescribed NSAID. These are preventable deaths, and they are prevented by the prescriber who checks interactions before signing the prescription. This chapter provides the quick-reference interaction tables organized for clinical speed.

24.1 CYP450 Master Reference

The CYP450 interaction system was introduced in section 2.2. These tables organize the information for rapid clinical lookup. When you are about to prescribe a medication, you need to answer two questions: (1) Which CYP enzymes metabolize this medication? (2) Does anything else in the patient's regimen inhibit or induce those enzymes?

CYP2D6 substrates (medications whose levels increase when a CYP2D6 inhibitor is added): aripiprazole, brexpiprazole, risperidone, haloperidol, perphenazine, fluoxetine, paroxetine, fluvoxamine, venlafaxine (to active metabolite), nortriptyline, desipramine, amitriptyline, atomoxetine, codeine (prodrug, will not activate), tramadol (prodrug, will not fully activate), dextromethorphan. **CYP2D6 potent inhibitors** (medications that increase levels of CYP2D6 substrates): fluoxetine, paroxetine, bupropion, quinidine. **CYP2D6 moderate inhibitors**: duloxetine, sertraline (at higher doses), terbinafine (Preskorn, 2013; Stahl, 2021).

The clinical translation: adding fluoxetine to a patient on aripiprazole will increase aripiprazole levels. The aripiprazole package insert recommends dose reduction to half the usual dose when co-prescribed with strong CYP2D6 inhibitors. Conversely, a patient who is a CYP2D6 poor metabolizer (section 3.2) already has reduced enzyme activity, so adding a CYP2D6 inhibitor compounds the effect further.

CYP2C19 substrates: citalopram, escitalopram, sertraline (partial), diazepam, phenytoin, proton pump inhibitors (omeprazole, esomeprazole, lansoprazole). **CYP2C19 inhibitors**: fluvoxamine (potent), fluoxetine (moderate), omeprazole (moderate). The clinical relevance: a CYP2C19 poor metabolizer on citalopram accumulates higher levels with increased QTc risk. The FDA maximum citalopram dose for CYP2C19 poor metabolizers is 20mg daily (Hicks et al., 2015).

CYP3A4 substrates: quetiapine, lurasidone, buspirone, alprazolam, midazolam, triazolam, carbamazepine (auto-inducer), pimozide, ziprasidone. **CYP3A4 potent inhibitors**: ketoconazole, itraconazole, clarithromycin, ritonavir, nefazodone, grapefruit juice. **CYP3A4 potent inducers**: carbamazepine, phenytoin, phenobarbital, rifampin, St. John's Wort. The clinical translation: a patient on quetiapine who starts carbamazepine will experience dramatically reduced quetiapine levels as CYP3A4 induction increases quetiapine metabolism. Quetiapine dose may need to increase 5-fold to maintain therapeutic levels, or an alternative antipsychotic should be selected (Stahl, 2021).

CYP1A2 substrates: clozapine, olanzapine, duloxetine, fluvoxamine, theophylline, caffeine. **CYP1A2 inducers**: smoking (polycyclic aromatic hydrocarbons, not nicotine), charbroiled foods, cruciferous vegetables (modest effect). **CYP1A2 potent inhibitor**: fluvoxamine. The clinical translation: a patient on clozapine who quits smoking will see clozapine levels rise 50-70% over 2-4 weeks. Dose reduction of approximately 25-50% should be initiated proactively when a clozapine patient quits smoking. Nicotine replacement therapy does not affect CYP1A2 because it is the smoke, not the nicotine, that induces the enzyme (Stahl, 2021).

24.2 QTc Prolongation Combinations

QTc prolongation becomes clinically dangerous when multiple prolonging agents are combined, when electrolyte abnormalities are present, or when the patient has underlying cardiac conduction disease.

High-risk psychotropic agents (significant independent QTc prolongation): thioridazine (greatest risk among antipsychotics, rarely used), ziprasidone, IV haloperidol (not oral haloperidol at standard doses), citalopram (dose-dependent, above 40mg), pimozide. **Moderate-risk agents** (modest independent QTc effect that becomes significant in combination): quetiapine, risperidone, olanzapine, chlorpromazine, escitalopram (at higher doses), TCAs.

When to obtain ECG: Before starting any high-risk agent. When combining two or more moderate-risk agents. When the patient has personal or family history of cardiac arrhythmia, syncope, or sudden death. When electrolyte abnormalities are present or likely (eating disorders, diuretic use, chronic vomiting). After dose increases of high-risk agents.

QTc thresholds: QTc above 500ms or increase of more than 60ms from baseline: immediate medication reassessment, cardiology consultation, electrolyte correction. QTc 470-500ms (males) or 480-500ms (females): risk-benefit reassessment, consider alternative agents, close monitoring. Normal QTc: below 440ms (males), below 460ms (females) (Beach et al., 2013).

24.3 Serotonergic Interaction Table

Serotonin syndrome risk is determined by the mechanism and potency of serotonergic activity in the combination.

Highest risk combinations (contraindicated or extreme caution): Any SSRI/SNRI + MAOI. Any SSRI/SNRI + linezolid (antibiotic with MAOI properties). Any SSRI/SNRI + methylene blue (IV, has MAOI properties). These combinations require mandatory washout periods: 14 days after discontinuing an MAOI before starting an SSRI/SNRI. 14 days after discontinuing most SSRIs/SNRIs before starting an MAOI. **5 weeks** after discontinuing fluoxetine before starting an MAOI (due to norfluoxetine's prolonged half-life) (Boyer & Shannon, 2005).

Moderate risk combinations (use with caution, monitor): SSRI/SNRI + tramadol (serotonin reuptake inhibition plus direct serotonergic activity). SSRI/SNRI + triptans (direct 5-HT1 agonism; risk is lower than previously believed, but monitoring is warranted). SSRI/SNRI + lithium (lithium enhances serotonergic transmission). SSRI + buspirone (additive 5-HT1A agonism; generally well tolerated). High-dose SSRI/SNRI monotherapy (serotonin syndrome can occur rarely at very high doses or in susceptible individuals).

Lower risk combinations (generally acceptable with awareness): SSRI + mirtazapine (different mechanisms, commonly combined as "California rocket fuel"). SSRI + trazodone (commonly used for insomnia augmentation). These are routine clinical combinations, but the prescriber should be aware that serotonergic activity is being enhanced.

24.4 Controlled Substance Reference

Controlled substance prescribing in psychiatric practice involves Schedule II through V medications with varying regulatory requirements.

Schedule II (highest abuse potential among prescribed medications, no refills, e-prescribing mandated in most states): amphetamine formulations (Adderall, Vyvanse, Dexedrine), methylphenidate formulations (Ritalin, Concerta, Focalin), methadone (when prescribed for pain; OTP regulations differ). **Schedule III**: buprenorphine/naloxone (Suboxone, X-waiver eliminated in 2023), esketamine (Spravato, REMS-mandated clinic administration), testosterone. **Schedule IV**: benzodiazepines (alprazolam, clonazepam, lorazepam, diazepam), Z-drugs (zolpidem, zaleplon, eszopiclone), modafinil, suvorexant. **Schedule V**: pregabalin (reclassified in some states), lacosamide, certain cough preparations (Stahl, 2021).

PDMP (Prescription Drug Monitoring Program) requirements vary by state but generally mandate checking the database before prescribing or dispensing Schedule II-IV controlled substances. Most states require a check at initial prescription and at intervals of 3-12 months thereafter. PDMP checking is a clinical best practice for all controlled substance prescriptions and is now a legal requirement in the majority of US states.

Prescribing documentation for controlled substances should include: the specific indication, prior treatment history (non-controlled alternatives tried), risk assessment for misuse (personal and family SUD history), informed consent regarding risks and monitoring expectations, and a clear plan for duration and reassessment intervals.

24.5 Clinical Implications

Drug interaction awareness is not a luxury of careful prescribers. It is a minimum standard of safe practice. The CYP450 tables in this chapter should be consulted whenever a medication is added to or removed from a patient's regimen. The QTc reference should be checked whenever a QTc-prolonging agent is prescribed. The serotonergic interaction table should be reviewed whenever combining serotonergic agents. And controlled substance regulations should be verified for each state in which the prescriber practices, because requirements change more frequently than any textbook can track.

25.1 Baseline Assessment Checklists

Universal baseline for all new psychiatric patients (regardless of medication planned): weight, BMI, blood pressure, heart rate, mental status examination, suicide risk screening (C-SSRS), substance use screening (AUDIT-C), pregnancy status for reproductive-age patients, current medication list with OTC and supplements. This assessment takes under 10 minutes and should be documented before any new medication is prescribed (American Diabetes Association et al., 2004).

SSRI/SNRI initiation: Universal baseline above. No additional labs required for most patients. Exceptions: baseline ECG if prescribing citalopram above 20mg or if patient is over 60. Baseline sodium if patient is elderly (SSRIs can cause hyponatremia via SIADH). Baseline hepatic function if prescribing duloxetine. Blood pressure if prescribing venlafaxine or desvenlafaxine (dose-dependent hypertension risk) (Stahl, 2021).

Atypical antipsychotic initiation: Universal baseline plus fasting glucose, fasting lipid panel (total cholesterol, LDL, HDL, triglycerides), HbA1c, waist circumference, baseline ECG (for ziprasidone or if risk factors present). These metabolic parameters form the monitoring foundation described by the APA/ADA consensus guidelines. The investment in baseline metabolic data pays dividends for years: without it, you cannot distinguish medication-induced metabolic changes from pre-existing conditions (American Diabetes Association et al., 2004).

Lithium initiation: Universal baseline plus serum creatinine and BUN (renal function), eGFR, TSH (thyroid function), calcium, ECG, pregnancy test for reproductive-age patients. These reflect lithium's primary organ toxicities: renal (nephrogenic diabetes insipidus, chronic interstitial nephritis), thyroid (hypothyroidism in 5-35% of patients), parathyroid (hyperparathyroidism with hypercalcemia), and cardiac (T-wave changes, sinus node dysfunction) (Malhi et al., 2017).

Valproate initiation: Universal baseline plus hepatic function panel (AST, ALT, total bilirubin), CBC with platelets, pregnancy test for reproductive-age patients. Valproate is hepatotoxic (rarely, but fatally in susceptible individuals, primarily children under 2 with mitochondrial disorders), causes thrombocytopenia at higher levels, and is the highest-teratogenicity-risk medication in psychiatric prescribing (Stahl, 2021).

Clozapine initiation: Universal baseline plus ANC (must be at least 1500/mcL, or 1000/mcL with documented benign ethnic neutropenia), fasting glucose, fasting lipid panel, HbA1c, hepatic function, ECG. Following the 2025 REMS elimination, the ANC monitoring schedule remains clinically required even though the centralized database and dispense authorization requirements have been removed (Stahl, 2021).

Carbamazepine initiation: Universal baseline plus CBC with differential, hepatic function, sodium, HLA-B*1502 (if Southeast Asian descent) and HLA-A*3101 (recommended for broader populations). Carbamazepine causes aplastic anemia and agranulocytosis (rare but serious), hyponatremia (SIADH), hepatotoxicity, and Stevens-Johnson syndrome in HLA-positive individuals (Leckband et al., 2013).

Lamotrigine initiation: No specific baseline labs required beyond universal assessment. The monitoring for lamotrigine is clinical, not laboratory: patient education about rash recognition (any new rash during titration should prompt immediate clinical contact), strict adherence to the titration schedule, and halved titration when co-prescribed with valproate (section 6.3).

25.2 Ongoing Monitoring Schedules

Atypical antipsychotic metabolic monitoring follows the APA/ADA consensus timeline:

Weight: baseline, 4 weeks, 8 weeks, 12 weeks, then quarterly. A weight gain of 7% or more from baseline at any point triggers clinical action (lifestyle intervention, consider medication switch, consider metformin). Blood pressure: baseline and at 12 weeks. Fasting glucose: baseline, 12 weeks, then annually. Fasting lipid panel: baseline, 12 weeks, then every 5 years (annually for patients with elevated baseline or on highest-risk agents like olanzapine or clozapine). HbA1c: baseline and annually. Waist circumference: baseline and annually (American Diabetes Association et al., 2004).

Lithium monitoring: Lithium level 5-7 days after initiation or any dose change (trough level, drawn 12 hours post-dose). Target range: 0.6-1.2 mEq/L for acute treatment, 0.6-0.8 mEq/L for maintenance. After stabilization: lithium level every 3 months for the first year, then every 6 months. Renal function (creatinine, eGFR): every 6 months. TSH: every 6 months. Calcium: annually. More frequent monitoring if clinically indicated (new medications, illness, dehydration, dose changes) (Malhi et al., 2017).

Valproate monitoring: Valproate level 3-5 days after initiation or dose change. Target range: 50-125 mcg/mL for acute mania (higher end), 50-100 mcg/mL for maintenance. Hepatic function: monthly for the first 6 months, then every 6-12 months. CBC with platelets: every 6-12 months (thrombocytopenia is dose-related). Ammonia level: check if the patient develops unexplained lethargy, confusion, or vomiting (hyperammonemia can occur even with normal hepatic function tests) (Stahl, 2021).

Clozapine ANC monitoring: Weekly for the first 6 months. Biweekly for months 6 through 12. Monthly thereafter for the duration of treatment. ANC thresholds for action: ANC below 1500/mcL in the general population (below 1000 in benign ethnic neutropenia): withhold clozapine and monitor daily until ANC recovers. ANC below 500: discontinue clozapine, do not rechallenge. Additional clozapine monitoring: fasting glucose and lipids at 12 weeks and annually; clozapine level at steady state (target 350-420 ng/mL for optimal response); ECG at baseline and if cardiac symptoms develop (Stahl, 2021).

Carbamazepine monitoring: CBC with differential at baseline, monthly for the first 2 months, then every 6-12 months. Sodium at baseline and periodically (watch for hyponatremia). Carbamazepine level for therapeutic monitoring (target 4-12 mcg/mL for seizure disorders; levels are less standardized for psychiatric indications but help assess adherence and toxicity risk). Hepatic function periodically (Stahl, 2021).

Consider the case of Kavya (composite example), a 45-year-old woman with bipolar I disorder initiated on lithium 600mg twice daily and quetiapine 300mg at bedtime 3 months ago. She presents for routine monitoring. The monitoring checklist: lithium level (drawn this morning as a trough, 12 hours post-dose): 0.72 mEq/L (therapeutic). Creatinine: 0.9 (stable from baseline). TSH: 5.2 mIU/L (elevated from baseline of 2.1, indicating lithium-induced subclinical hypothyroidism). Fasting glucose: 104 (borderline, increased from baseline of 88). Weight: up 8 pounds from baseline (5.3% increase, approaching the 7% clinical action threshold). The clinical actions: (1) Initiate levothyroxine 25mcg daily for subclinical hypothyroidism, recheck TSH in 6-8 weeks. (2) Intensify lifestyle counseling for metabolic changes. (3) Recheck fasting glucose and HbA1c at 6-month visit. (4) Continue lithium and quetiapine but monitor weight closely, with a plan to consider quetiapine alternatives if weight gain exceeds 7%. This routine monitoring visit detected two developing problems (thyroid and metabolic) early enough for intervention.

25.3 Rating Scale Quick Reference

Standardized rating scales were introduced in section 4.1 and are used throughout the diagnosis-based chapters for treatment response tracking. This section consolidates scoring, interpretation, and clinical action thresholds for rapid reference.

PHQ-9 (Patient Health Questionnaire-9): 9 items scored 0-3 each. Total range: 0-27. Severity: 0-4 minimal, 5-9 mild, 10-14 moderate, 15-19 moderately severe, 20-27 severe. Response: 50% or greater reduction from baseline. Remission: score below 5. Clinical action: administer at every medication visit; scores guide dose optimization, augmentation, and treatment resistance determination. Item 9 (suicidal ideation) requires follow-up with structured risk assessment if endorsed (Kroenke et al., 2001).

GAD-7 (Generalized Anxiety Disorder-7): 7 items scored 0-3 each. Total range: 0-21. Severity: 0-4 minimal, 5-9 mild, 10-14 moderate, 15-21 severe. Response: 50% or greater reduction. Remission: score below 5. Clinical action: administer at every medication visit for anxiety disorders; guides anxiolytic dose optimization and augmentation decisions (Spitzer et al., 2006).

MDQ (Mood Disorder Questionnaire): 13 yes/no items in Part 1, plus questions about symptom co-occurrence and functional impairment. Positive screen: 7+ yes responses in Part 1, symptoms occurring together, and causing moderate-to-serious functional impairment. Clinical action: a positive screen does not diagnose bipolar disorder but prompts further clinical assessment before initiating antidepressant monotherapy (Hirschfeld et al., 2000).

PCL-5 (PTSD Checklist for DSM-5): 20 items scored 0-4 each. Total range: 0-80. Provisional PTSD diagnosis: score of 31-33 or above (varies by setting and population). Clinically meaningful change: 10-point decrease from baseline. Clinical action: administer monthly during PTSD treatment; guides prazosin titration for nightmares and SSRI optimization for daytime symptoms (Bovin et al., 2016).

C-SSRS (Columbia Suicide Severity Rating Scale): Structured interview assessing suicidal ideation intensity, behavior, and lethality. Categories: no ideation, passive ideation ("wish I were dead"), active ideation without plan, active ideation with plan, active ideation with intent, preparatory behavior, actual attempt. Clinical action: administer at every medication visit. Any endorsement of active ideation with plan or above triggers immediate safety assessment and intervention. Document the C-SSRS category at every visit (Posner et al., 2011).

ASRS (Adult ADHD Self-Report Scale): 6-item screener version. Part A: 6 items scored on frequency scale. 4+ items in the shaded area suggest further evaluation. Clinical action: screen adults presenting with attention and concentration complaints before diagnosing ADHD and prescribing stimulants. The full 18-item version provides more detailed symptom tracking for treatment monitoring (Kessler et al., 2005).

25.4 Synthesis

Monitoring transforms prescribing from a one-time decision into an ongoing clinical process. Baseline assessments establish the reference point from which all changes are measured. Ongoing monitoring schedules are medication-class-specific and must be followed systematically. Rating scales provide the objective symptom data that anchors prescribing decisions to measurable outcomes. When monitoring detects a problem (rising lithium levels, metabolic deterioration, worsening depression scores, emerging suicidal ideation), the clinical response is immediate and documented. When monitoring confirms stability, it supports the decision to maintain the current regimen. Either way, the data drives the decision.

Chapter 25.0: Monitoring Parameter Reference

Monitoring is not documentation for liability protection. Monitoring is the clinical mechanism by which you detect medication toxicity before it harms your patient, confirm therapeutic response with objective data, and make informed decisions about dose adjustments and treatment changes. Every monitoring parameter in this chapter has a clinical action threshold, a frequency interval, and a rationale. If you cannot articulate why you are ordering a lab, you probably should not order it. And if a lab is indicated but not ordered, you have missed a safety obligation.

25.1 Baseline Assessment Checklists

Universal baseline for all new psychiatric patients (regardless of medication planned): weight, BMI, blood pressure, heart rate, mental status examination, suicide risk screening (C-SSRS), substance use screening (AUDIT-C), pregnancy status for reproductive-age patients, current medication list with OTC and supplements. This assessment takes under 10 minutes and should be documented before any new medication is prescribed (American Diabetes Association et al., 2004).

SSRI/SNRI initiation: Universal baseline above. No additional labs required for most patients. Exceptions: baseline ECG if prescribing citalopram above 20mg or if patient is over 60. Baseline sodium if patient is elderly (SSRIs can cause hyponatremia via SIADH). Baseline hepatic function if prescribing duloxetine. Blood pressure if prescribing venlafaxine or desvenlafaxine (dose-dependent hypertension risk) (Stahl, 2021).

Atypical antipsychotic initiation: Universal baseline plus fasting glucose, fasting lipid panel (total cholesterol, LDL, HDL, triglycerides), HbA1c, waist circumference, baseline ECG (for ziprasidone or if risk factors present). These metabolic parameters form the monitoring foundation described by the APA/ADA consensus guidelines. The investment in baseline metabolic data pays dividends for years: without it, you cannot distinguish medication-induced metabolic changes from pre-existing conditions (American Diabetes Association et al., 2004).

Lithium initiation: Universal baseline plus serum creatinine and BUN (renal function), eGFR, TSH (thyroid function), calcium, ECG, pregnancy test for reproductive-age patients. These reflect lithium's primary organ toxicities: renal (nephrogenic diabetes insipidus, chronic interstitial nephritis), thyroid (hypothyroidism in 5-35% of patients), parathyroid (hyperparathyroidism with hypercalcemia), and cardiac (T-wave changes, sinus node dysfunction) (Malhi et al., 2017).

Valproate initiation: Universal baseline plus hepatic function panel (AST, ALT, total bilirubin), CBC with platelets, pregnancy test for reproductive-age patients. Valproate is hepatotoxic (rarely, but fatally in susceptible individuals, primarily children under 2 with mitochondrial disorders), causes thrombocytopenia at higher levels, and is the highest-teratogenicity-risk medication in psychiatric prescribing (Stahl, 2021).

Clozapine initiation: Universal baseline plus ANC (must be at least 1500/mcL, or 1000/mcL with documented benign ethnic neutropenia), fasting glucose, fasting lipid panel, HbA1c, hepatic function, ECG. Following the 2025 REMS elimination, the ANC monitoring schedule remains clinically required even though the centralized database and dispense authorization requirements have been removed (Stahl, 2021).

Carbamazepine initiation: Universal baseline plus CBC with differential, hepatic function, sodium, HLA-B*1502 (if Southeast Asian descent) and HLA-A*3101 (recommended for broader populations). Carbamazepine causes aplastic anemia and agranulocytosis (rare but serious), hyponatremia (SIADH), hepatotoxicity, and Stevens-Johnson syndrome in HLA-positive individuals (Leckband et al., 2013).

Lamotrigine initiation: No specific baseline labs required beyond universal assessment. The monitoring for lamotrigine is clinical, not laboratory: patient education about rash recognition (any new rash during titration should prompt immediate clinical contact), strict adherence to the titration schedule, and halved titration when co-prescribed with valproate (section 6.3).

25.2 Ongoing Monitoring Schedules

Atypical antipsychotic metabolic monitoring follows the APA/ADA consensus timeline:

Weight: baseline, 4 weeks, 8 weeks, 12 weeks, then quarterly. A weight gain of 7% or more from baseline at any point triggers clinical action (lifestyle intervention, consider medication switch, consider metformin). Blood pressure: baseline and at 12 weeks. Fasting glucose: baseline, 12 weeks, then annually. Fasting lipid panel: baseline, 12 weeks, then every 5 years (annually for patients with elevated baseline or on highest-risk agents like olanzapine or clozapine). HbA1c: baseline and annually. Waist circumference: baseline and annually (American Diabetes Association et al., 2004).

Lithium monitoring: Lithium level 5-7 days after initiation or any dose change (trough level, drawn 12 hours post-dose). Target range: 0.6-1.2 mEq/L for acute treatment, 0.6-0.8 mEq/L for maintenance. After stabilization: lithium level every 3 months for the first year, then every 6 months. Renal function (creatinine, eGFR): every 6 months. TSH: every 6 months. Calcium: annually. More frequent monitoring if clinically indicated (new medications, illness, dehydration, dose changes) (Malhi et al., 2017).

Valproate monitoring: Valproate level 3-5 days after initiation or dose change. Target range: 50-125 mcg/mL for acute mania (higher end), 50-100 mcg/mL for maintenance. Hepatic function: monthly for the first 6 months, then every 6-12 months. CBC with platelets: every 6-12 months (thrombocytopenia is dose-related). Ammonia level: check if the patient develops unexplained lethargy, confusion, or vomiting (hyperammonemia can occur even with normal hepatic function tests) (Stahl, 2021).

Clozapine ANC monitoring: Weekly for the first 6 months. Biweekly for months 6 through 12. Monthly thereafter for the duration of treatment. ANC thresholds for action: ANC below 1500/mcL in the general population (below 1000 in benign ethnic neutropenia): withhold clozapine and monitor daily until ANC recovers. ANC below 500: discontinue clozapine, do not rechallenge. Additional clozapine monitoring: fasting glucose and lipids at 12 weeks and annually; clozapine level at steady state (target 350-420 ng/mL for optimal response); ECG at baseline and if cardiac symptoms develop (Stahl, 2021).

Carbamazepine monitoring: CBC with differential at baseline, monthly for the first 2 months, then every 6-12 months. Sodium at baseline and periodically (watch for hyponatremia). Carbamazepine level for therapeutic monitoring (target 4-12 mcg/mL for seizure disorders; levels are less standardized for psychiatric indications but help assess adherence and toxicity risk). Hepatic function periodically (Stahl, 2021).

Consider the case of Kavya (composite example), a 45-year-old woman with bipolar I disorder initiated on lithium 600mg twice daily and quetiapine 300mg at bedtime 3 months ago. She presents for routine monitoring. The monitoring checklist: lithium level (drawn this morning as a trough, 12 hours post-dose): 0.72 mEq/L (therapeutic). Creatinine: 0.9 (stable from baseline). TSH: 5.2 mIU/L (elevated from baseline of 2.1, indicating lithium-induced subclinical hypothyroidism). Fasting glucose: 104 (borderline, increased from baseline of 88). Weight: up 8 pounds from baseline (5.3% increase, approaching the 7% clinical action threshold). The clinical actions: (1) Initiate levothyroxine 25mcg daily for subclinical hypothyroidism, recheck TSH in 6-8 weeks. (2) Intensify lifestyle counseling for metabolic changes. (3) Recheck fasting glucose and HbA1c at 6-month visit. (4) Continue lithium and quetiapine but monitor weight closely, with a plan to consider quetiapine alternatives if weight gain exceeds 7%. This routine monitoring visit detected two developing problems (thyroid and metabolic) early enough for intervention.

25.4 Synthesis

Monitoring transforms prescribing from a one-time decision into an ongoing clinical process. Baseline assessments establish the reference point from which all changes are measured. Ongoing monitoring schedules are medication-class-specific and must be followed systematically. Rating scales provide the objective symptom data that anchors prescribing decisions to measurable outcomes. When monitoring detects a problem (rising lithium levels, metabolic deterioration, worsening depression scores, emerging suicidal ideation), the clinical response is immediate and documented. When monitoring confirms stability, it supports the decision to maintain the current regimen. Either way, the data drives the decision.

Chapter 26.0: Patient Education and Decisions

The best prescribing decision means nothing if the patient does not take the medication. Nonadherence rates for psychiatric medications range from 20% to 60% depending on the diagnosis, medication class, and population studied. The reasons are predictable: side effects, stigma, lack of understanding about why the medication works, unrealistic expectations about onset of action, and cultural factors that influence attitudes toward psychiatric treatment. This chapter addresses the prescriber's role in patient education, informed consent, and shared decision-making as clinical skills that are as consequential as medication selection itself.

26.1 Medication Education Frameworks

The **teach-back method** is the most effective technique for confirming patient understanding. After explaining a medication, ask the patient to repeat back in their own words: what the medication is for, how to take it, what side effects to watch for, and when to contact the clinic. This is not a test of the patient's intelligence. It is a test of the prescriber's communication clarity. If the patient cannot teach it back, the explanation was insufficient (Schillinger et al., 2003).

Setting expectations for onset of action prevents premature discontinuation. Patients starting SSRIs need to know: "You may notice some side effects (nausea, headache, sleep changes) in the first week. These usually improve within 7-10 days. The antidepressant effect takes 2-4 weeks to begin and 6-8 weeks to reach full effect. If you stop taking the medication after one week because you don't feel better, you haven't given it enough time to work." This specific framing reduces early dropout (Stahl, 2021).

Side effect counseling should be honest and specific. Rather than listing every possible side effect from the package insert (which overwhelms patients and increases nocebo effects), focus on the 2-3 most likely side effects for that specific patient's medication, explain what they feel like, and describe what to do if they occur. For sertraline: "The most common early side effects are nausea and loose stools, which usually improve within 1-2 weeks. Some patients notice changes in sexual function after a few weeks. If any side effect is bothering you, call us before stopping the medication, because we often have ways to manage it."

Addressing stigma requires direct conversation, not avoidance. Many patients resist psychiatric medication because they perceive it as a sign of weakness, a crutch, or a life sentence. The prescriber's role is to normalize pharmacotherapy within the broader context of medical treatment: "We use medication to treat the neurobiological component of depression the same way we use medication for the biological component of diabetes or hypertension. It doesn't mean you're weak. It means your brain chemistry needs support while you do the work of therapy and recovery" (Corrigan et al., 2014).

26.2 Informed Consent Essentials

Informed consent for psychiatric medication is not a form to be signed. It is a conversation to be documented. The legal and ethical requirements include: the nature of the condition being treated, the proposed medication and its mechanism, the expected benefits and timeline, the material risks and common side effects, the alternatives to the proposed medication (including no medication), and the patient's questions and the prescriber's responses.

Specific consent conversations are warranted for higher-risk medications. **Clozapine**: discuss the risk of severe neutropenia, the monitoring schedule, symptoms requiring immediate medical attention (fever, sore throat, flu-like illness), metabolic effects, sedation, constipation management, and seizure risk. **Lithium**: discuss the narrow therapeutic window, the importance of consistent hydration, medications to avoid (NSAIDs, dehydration), the need for regular blood monitoring, and symptoms of toxicity (tremor worsening, confusion, vomiting, diarrhea). **MAOIs**: discuss dietary tyramine restriction, the list of medications that must be avoided, and symptoms of hypertensive crisis (severe headache, stiff neck, nausea). **Controlled substances**: discuss the risk of dependence, the legal requirements around prescription management, and the agreement regarding monitoring expectations (Stahl, 2021).

Consider the case of Layla (composite example), a 41-year-old woman with treatment-resistant depression who has been recommended esketamine (Spravato). The informed consent conversation covers: the REMS requirements (clinic-based administration, 2-hour observation period), the expected experience during administration (dissociation, dizziness, altered perception that resolves within 1-2 hours), the treatment schedule (twice weekly for 4 weeks, then weekly for 4 weeks, then weekly or biweekly as maintenance), the common side effects (nausea, dizziness, dissociation, sedation, increased blood pressure during administration), the requirement that she arrange transportation home after each session (she cannot drive for the remainder of the day), and the fact that response typically begins within 24 hours of the first dose but that multiple sessions are needed for sustained improvement. She asks if the dissociation feels like being "high." The prescriber explains that some patients find the dissociation unpleasant, others neutral, and a few pleasant, but that the therapeutic mechanism does not depend on the subjective experience of dissociation. Her questions are answered. Consent is documented. Treatment begins.

26.3 Shared Decision-Making

Shared decision-making (SDM) is the process of integrating clinical evidence with patient values and preferences to arrive at a mutually agreed-upon treatment plan. It is not the prescriber dictating a plan, and it is not the patient choosing medications from a menu. It is a dialogue in which the prescriber contributes clinical expertise and the patient contributes knowledge of their own life, values, and priorities (Deegan & Drake, 2006).

Practical SDM in a 15-minute medication visit looks like this: "Based on your symptoms and what you've told me about your priorities, I see two reasonable options. We could try duloxetine, which addresses both your depression and your chronic pain but might cause some nausea initially. Or we could try bupropion, which is less likely to cause sexual side effects and might help with your energy, but it won't help your pain. Both have good evidence. What matters most to you right now?"

When patient preference conflicts with clinical judgment: This occurs most commonly when patients request benzodiazepines for anxiety when SSRIs would be more appropriate, or when patients refuse a recommended medication based on stigma or misinformation. The prescriber's obligation is to explain the clinical reasoning, provide accurate information, and respect the patient's autonomy while documenting the discussion. "I understand you'd prefer a medication that works immediately, and I hear that the anxiety is difficult to tolerate. Benzodiazepines provide quick relief but create dependence and don't address the underlying problem. An SSRI takes longer to work but provides sustained relief without dependence. I'd like to start the SSRI today and give you hydroxyzine for the worst anxiety moments while we wait for the SSRI to take effect. Would that be an acceptable plan?"

Cultural considerations in prescribing extend beyond language translation. Some cultures view psychiatric medication as shameful. Some prioritize family decision-making over individual autonomy. Some have traditional healing practices that patients use concurrently with Western medication (with potential interaction risks). The culturally competent prescriber asks about these factors directly: "Are there any cultural or family considerations that affect how you feel about taking this medication? Are you using any traditional remedies or supplements I should know about?" (Corrigan et al., 2014).

Consider the case of Hassan (composite example), a 55-year-old man with bipolar I disorder who has been stable on lithium for 8 years. He presents reporting that he wants to stop lithium because he "feels fine now" and believes he no longer needs it. The SDM conversation acknowledges his perspective while providing the clinical context: "I understand the desire to stop a medication when you're feeling well. That's a reasonable question. Here's what the evidence tells us: after 8 years of stability on lithium, stopping it carries a relapse risk of 50-90% within the first year, and relapse often occurs within weeks to months. Lithium also has unique properties that reduce suicide risk, which is meaningful given your history. The trade-off is continued monitoring and the side effects you experience. What if we discussed what's bothering you about lithium? If it's the blood draws, we could reduce the frequency. If it's a specific side effect, we might be able to address it. Staying on a medication that's working well for you is something I'd strongly recommend, but I want to understand what's driving this request." The outcome: Hassan reveals that a coworker told him lithium causes permanent kidney damage and he is frightened. The prescriber addresses the concern with accurate information about lithium nephrotoxicity (rare with proper monitoring, his renal function has been stable for 8 years) and the conversation shifts from discontinuation to ongoing monitoring reassurance.

26.4 Summary and Recommendations

Patient education, informed consent, and shared decision-making are clinical skills that directly affect medication adherence, treatment outcomes, and patient safety. The teach-back method confirms understanding. Setting realistic expectations about onset and side effects prevents premature discontinuation. Informed consent conversations are most critical for higher-risk medications (clozapine, lithium, MAOIs, controlled substances, esketamine). Shared decision-making respects patient autonomy while ensuring that clinical evidence informs the choice. Cultural humility requires asking about beliefs and practices that may affect medication acceptance and adherence. The prescriber who invests 2-3 minutes in education at the point of prescribing saves hours of managing the consequences of nonadherence, premature discontinuation, and miscommunication.

Appendices

Appendix A: Dosing Quick Reference

This appendix consolidates starting doses, therapeutic ranges, maximum doses, and approximate half-lives for the psychiatric medications most commonly prescribed by PMHNPs and advanced practice providers. Doses listed are for adults unless otherwise noted. Geriatric dosing generally starts at 50% of the listed starting dose (section 20.1). Pediatric dosing follows age-specific guidelines in Chapter 19.0. Pharmacogenomic considerations (section 3.2) and hepatic/renal impairment (sections 21.1 and 21.2) may require further adjustment. All information reflects FDA-approved labeling and established clinical practice as of 2025.

A.1 Antidepressant Dosing

Selective Serotonin Reuptake Inhibitors (SSRIs)

Sertraline (Zoloft): Starting dose 50mg daily. Therapeutic range 50-200mg. Maximum 200mg. Half-life approximately 26 hours. Clinical notes: generally weight-neutral, mild dopaminergic activity, broad evidence base across depression subtypes. Start at 25mg for panic disorder.

Escitalopram (Lexapro): Starting dose 10mg daily. Therapeutic range 10-20mg. Maximum 20mg. Half-life approximately 27-32 hours. Clinical notes: cleanest pharmacology among SSRIs, fewest drug interactions, preferred in medically complex patients. CYP2C19 poor metabolizers: maximum 10mg.

Fluoxetine (Prozac): Starting dose 20mg daily. Therapeutic range 20-80mg. Maximum 80mg. Half-life 1-3 days (active metabolite norfluoxetine: 4-16 days). Clinical notes: longest half-life, least discontinuation syndrome, potent CYP2D6 inhibitor, activating. Requires 5-week washout before MAOI.

Citalopram (Celexa): Starting dose 20mg daily. Therapeutic range 20-40mg. Maximum 40mg (20mg if age 60+, hepatic impairment, or CYP2C19 poor metabolizer). Half-life approximately 35 hours. Clinical notes: dose-dependent QTc prolongation, FDA dose ceiling.

Paroxetine (Paxil): Starting dose 20mg daily. Therapeutic range 20-60mg. Maximum 60mg. Half-life approximately 21 hours. Clinical notes: most sedating SSRI, highest sexual dysfunction rate, highest weight gain, potent CYP2D6 inhibitor, significant discontinuation syndrome. Generally not preferred as first-line.

Fluvoxamine (Luvox): Starting dose 50mg daily. Therapeutic range 100-300mg. Maximum 300mg. Half-life approximately 15 hours. Clinical notes: primarily used for OCD, potent CYP1A2 inhibitor (avoid with clozapine, olanzapine).

Serotonin-Norepinephrine Reuptake Inhibitors (SNRIs)

Venlafaxine XR (Effexor XR): Starting dose 37.5-75mg daily. Therapeutic range 75-225mg. Maximum 225mg (375mg in some guidelines). Half-life approximately 5 hours (active metabolite O-desmethylvenlafaxine: 11 hours). Clinical notes: primarily serotonergic below 150mg, adds norepinephrine above 150mg, monitor blood pressure, significant discontinuation syndrome.

Duloxetine (Cymbalta): Starting dose 30mg daily for 1 week, then 60mg. Therapeutic range 60-120mg. Maximum 120mg. Half-life approximately 12 hours. Clinical notes: FDA-approved for MDD, GAD, diabetic neuropathy, fibromyalgia, chronic musculoskeletal pain. Contraindicated in substantial alcohol use or chronic liver disease.

Desvenlafaxine (Pristiq): Starting dose 50mg daily. Therapeutic range 50mg. Maximum 100mg (minimal additional benefit above 50mg). Half-life approximately 11 hours. Clinical notes: active metabolite of venlafaxine, less CYP-dependent metabolism, requires dose adjustment in severe renal impairment.

Levomilnacipran (Fetzima): Starting dose 20mg daily for 2 days, then 40mg. Therapeutic range 40-120mg. Maximum 120mg. Half-life approximately 12 hours. Clinical notes: preferential norepinephrine reuptake inhibition, may be useful for fatigue-predominant depression.

Other Antidepressants

Bupropion XL (Wellbutrin XL): Starting dose 150mg daily. Therapeutic range 150-450mg. Maximum 450mg. Half-life approximately 21 hours. Clinical notes: dopamine/norepinephrine mechanism, no serotonergic activity, no sexual dysfunction, seizure risk above 450mg, contraindicated in eating disorders and seizure disorders.

Mirtazapine (Remeron): Starting dose 15mg at bedtime. Therapeutic range 15-45mg. Maximum 45mg. Half-life approximately 20-40 hours. Clinical notes: sedation and appetite stimulation via H1 and 5-HT2C blockade, paradoxically less sedating at higher doses as noradrenergic activity increases.

Trazodone (Desyrel): Antidepressant dose 150-400mg. Insomnia dose 25-100mg at bedtime. Maximum 400mg. Half-life approximately 7-10 hours. Clinical notes: primarily used off-label for insomnia at low doses, priapism risk (rare but requires patient education).

Auvelity (dextromethorphan/bupropion): Starting dose 45mg/105mg daily for 3 days, then twice daily. Maximum 45mg/105mg twice daily. Clinical notes: NMDA antagonist mechanism, approved for MDD including treatment-resistant presentations.

A.2 Antipsychotic Dosing

Atypical Antipsychotics

Aripiprazole (Abilify): Starting dose 10-15mg daily. Therapeutic range 10-30mg. Maximum 30mg. Half-life approximately 75 hours. Clinical notes: D2 partial agonist, weight-neutral, minimal prolactin elevation, akathisia is primary limiting side effect. MDD augmentation dose: 2-15mg.

Quetiapine (Seroquel/Seroquel XR): Starting dose 25-50mg at bedtime (schizophrenia), 50mg at bedtime (bipolar depression). Therapeutic range 150-800mg. Maximum 800mg. Half-life approximately 7 hours. Clinical notes: sedation and metabolic effects dose-dependent, bipolar depression dose 300mg, insomnia dose 25-100mg (off-label). Metabolized by CYP3A4.

Risperidone (Risperdal): Starting dose 1-2mg daily. Therapeutic range 2-8mg. Maximum 16mg. Half-life approximately 20 hours (including active metabolite paliperidone). Clinical notes: highest prolactin elevation among atypicals, EPS increases above 6mg, available as LAI.

Olanzapine (Zyprexa): Starting dose 5-10mg at bedtime. Therapeutic range 10-20mg. Maximum 20mg. Half-life approximately 30 hours. Clinical notes: highest metabolic risk (weight gain, diabetes, dyslipidemia), most effective for acute mania, sedating. CYP1A2 substrate (smoking interaction).

Ziprasidone (Geodon): Starting dose 20mg twice daily with food. Therapeutic range 80-160mg. Maximum 160mg. Half-life approximately 6-7 hours. Clinical notes: must take with at least 500 calories, weight-neutral, highest QTc prolongation risk among atypicals, requires baseline ECG.

Lurasidone (Latuda): Starting dose 40mg daily with food (at least 350 calories). Therapeutic range 40-160mg. Maximum 160mg. Half-life approximately 18 hours. Clinical notes: favorable metabolic profile, food requirement is absolute, FDA-approved for bipolar I depression. CYP3A4 substrate.

Cariprazine (Vraylar): Starting dose 1.5mg daily. Therapeutic range 1.5-6mg. Maximum 6mg. Half-life approximately 2-4 days (active metabolite: 2-3 weeks). Clinical notes: D3-preferring partial agonist, long active metabolite means effects persist weeks after discontinuation, approved for schizophrenia, bipolar mania, and bipolar depression.

Brexpiprazole (Rexulti): Starting dose 0.5-1mg daily. Therapeutic range 2-4mg. Maximum 4mg. Half-life approximately 91 hours. Clinical notes: D2 partial agonist similar to aripiprazole but with less akathisia, FDA-approved for MDD augmentation (1-3mg) and Alzheimer's agitation (2-3mg).

Paliperidone (Invega): Starting dose 6mg daily. Therapeutic range 3-12mg. Maximum 12mg. Half-life approximately 23 hours. Clinical notes: active metabolite of risperidone, primarily renally eliminated (minimal hepatic metabolism), requires renal dose adjustment. Available as monthly and 3-month LAI (Invega Sustenna, Invega Trinza).

Clozapine (Clozaril): Starting dose 12.5mg once or twice daily. Therapeutic range 300-450mg. Maximum 900mg. Half-life approximately 12 hours. Clinical notes: gold standard for treatment-resistant schizophrenia, ANC monitoring required (weekly for 6 months, biweekly months 6-12, monthly thereafter), REMS eliminated 2025 but clinical monitoring unchanged. Target level 350-420 ng/mL. CYP1A2 substrate (smoking interaction).

Cobenfy (xanomeline/trospium): Starting dose 50mg/20mg twice daily. Therapeutic dose 125mg/30mg twice daily. Maximum 125mg/30mg twice daily. Clinical notes: first non-dopaminergic antipsychotic, muscarinic M1/M4 agonist mechanism, favorable metabolic/EPS/prolactin profile, GI side effects primary concern.

Lumateperone (Caplyta): Dose 42mg daily. No titration needed. Half-life approximately 18 hours. Clinical notes: FDA-approved for schizophrenia, bipolar I depression, bipolar II depression (monotherapy or adjunct to lithium/valproate), and adjunctive MDD treatment (2025). Favorable metabolic profile.

A.3 Mood Stabilizer Dosing

Lithium (Lithobid, generic): Starting dose 300mg two or three times daily. Therapeutic level: acute mania 0.8-1.2 mEq/L, maintenance 0.6-0.8 mEq/L. Maximum dose guided by level. Half-life approximately 18-24 hours. Clinical notes: check level 5-7 days after any dose change (trough, 12 hours post-dose), renal/thyroid/calcium monitoring required, drug interactions with NSAIDs, ACE inhibitors, thiazides.

Valproate/Divalproex (Depakote): Starting dose 250mg two or three times daily, or loading dose 20-30 mg/kg/day for acute mania. Therapeutic level 50-125 mcg/mL. Maximum guided by level and tolerability. Half-life approximately 9-16 hours. Clinical notes: effective for mixed features and rapid cycling, highest teratogenicity risk among mood stabilizers, hepatic/hematologic monitoring required.

Lamotrigine (Lamictal): Starting dose 25mg daily for 2 weeks, then 50mg daily for 2 weeks, then 100mg daily for 1 week, target 200mg daily. With valproate: halve the titration (25mg every other day for 2 weeks). Therapeutic range 100-400mg. Half-life approximately 25 hours (shorter with enzyme inducers, longer with valproate). Clinical notes: Stevens-Johnson syndrome risk mandates strict titration adherence, preferred mood stabilizer in pregnancy, better for depression prevention than mania prevention.

Carbamazepine (Tegretol): Starting dose 200mg twice daily. Therapeutic level 4-12 mcg/mL. Maximum 1600mg daily. Half-life 25-65 hours initially, 12-17 hours at steady state (auto-induction).

Clinical notes: potent CYP3A4/2C9/1A2 inducer, HLA screening required before initiation, reduces oral contraceptive efficacy, drug interaction-dense.

Oxcarbazepine (Trileptal): Starting dose 300mg twice daily. Therapeutic range 600-2400mg. Maximum 2400mg. Half-life approximately 9 hours (active metabolite). Clinical notes: fewer drug interactions than carbamazepine, less auto-induction, hyponatremia risk, HLA-B*1502 screening recommended.

A.4 Anxiolytic and Hypnotic Dosing

Buspirone: Starting dose 5mg two or three times daily. Therapeutic range 15-60mg. Maximum 60mg. Half-life approximately 2-3 hours. Clinical notes: 5-HT1A partial agonist, no sedation, no dependence, 2-4 week onset.

Hydroxyzine: 25-100mg as needed, up to 4 times daily. Maximum 400mg. Half-life approximately 20 hours. Clinical notes: H1 antagonist, sedating, no dependence potential, useful as benzodiazepine alternative for acute anxiety.

Suvorexant (Belsomra): 10mg nightly (20mg if tolerated). Maximum 20mg. Half-life approximately 12 hours. Clinical notes: dual orexin receptor antagonist, no GABA mechanism, no dependence, next-day somnolence possible.

Lemborexant (Dayvigo): 5mg nightly (10mg if needed). Maximum 10mg. Half-life approximately 17-19 hours. Clinical notes: DORA, sleep onset and maintenance, no GABA mechanism.

Ramelteon (Rozerem): 8mg nightly, 30 minutes before bedtime. Maximum 8mg. Half-life approximately 1-2.6 hours. Clinical notes: melatonin MT1/MT2 agonist, targets sleep onset only, no dependence, no rebound, safe in elderly.

Low-dose doxepin (Silenor): 3-6mg at bedtime. Maximum 6mg. Half-life approximately 15 hours. Clinical notes: FDA-approved for sleep maintenance insomnia, selective H1 antagonism at this dose, no antidepressant effect.

A.5 ADHD Medication Dosing

Lisdexamfetamine (Vyvanse): Starting dose 30mg daily (adults). Therapeutic range 30-70mg. Maximum 70mg. Duration 12-14 hours. Clinical notes: prodrug, lower misuse potential, also FDA-approved for binge eating disorder.

Mixed amphetamine salts XR (Adderall XR): Starting dose 20mg daily (adults). Therapeutic range 20-60mg. Maximum 60mg. Duration 10-12 hours.

Methylphenidate ER (Concerta): Starting dose 18mg daily (adults). Therapeutic range 18-72mg. Maximum 72mg. Duration 10-12 hours. Clinical notes: osmotic release mechanism.

Atomoxetine (Strattera): Starting dose 40mg daily. Therapeutic range 40-100mg (weight-based: 1.2 mg/kg). Maximum 100mg. Half-life approximately 5 hours (22 hours in CYP2D6 poor metabolizers). Clinical notes: NRI, no abuse potential, 4-6 week onset, CYP2D6 substrate.

Guanfacine ER (Intuniv): Starting dose 1mg daily. Therapeutic range 1-4mg. Maximum 4mg (children), 7mg (adults). Half-life approximately 17 hours. Clinical notes: alpha-2 agonist, useful for ADHD with comorbid tics or aggression.

Viloxazine ER (Qelbree): Adult starting dose 200mg daily. Therapeutic range 200-600mg. Maximum 600mg. Clinical notes: NRI with serotonergic modulation, approved for children, adolescents, and adults.

A.6 Substance Use Disorder Dosing

Naltrexone oral (ReVia): 50mg daily. Clinical notes: for AUD and OUD (after complete opioid detoxification), contraindicated with current opioid use.

Naltrexone IM (Vivitrol): 380mg monthly injection. Clinical notes: eliminates daily adherence variability, requires 7-14 days opioid-free before first injection.

Buprenorphine/naloxone (Suboxone): Induction 2-8mg on day 1, target 16-24mg maintenance. Maximum 24mg. Clinical notes: X-waiver eliminated 2023, traditional or micro-induction protocols available.

Acamprosate (Campral): 666mg three times daily. Clinical notes: renally eliminated, no hepatic metabolism, preferred in hepatic impairment.

Varenicline (Chantix): 0.5mg daily for 3 days, 0.5mg twice daily for 4 days, then 1mg twice daily for 12 weeks. Clinical notes: most effective single agent for tobacco cessation.

Appendix B: Benzodiazepine Equivalency and Tapering

This appendix provides the equivalency conversions and tapering protocols referenced throughout the book, particularly in section 7.4 (benzodiazepine management) and section 20.5 (geriatric deprescribing). The 2025 Joint Clinical Practice Guideline on Benzodiazepine Tapering serves as the primary evidence source (Brunner et al., 2025).

B.1 Diazepam Equivalency Table

All equivalencies are approximate and should be used as starting points, not absolute conversions. Individual variation in metabolism, tolerance, and sensitivity means that clinical monitoring during conversion is mandatory.

Diazepam 10mg is approximately equivalent to: Alprazolam 0.5mg. Chlordiazepoxide 25mg. Clonazepam 0.5mg. Lorazepam 1mg. Oxazepam 15-30mg. Temazepam 15-20mg. Triazolam 0.25mg.

Half-life classifications: Ultra-short acting (triazolam: 1.5-5.5 hours). Short acting (alprazolam: 6-12 hours, lorazepam: 10-20 hours, oxazepam: 4-15 hours, temazepam: 8-22 hours). Long acting (clonazepam: 18-50 hours, diazepam: 20-100 hours including active metabolite desmethyldiazepam, chlordiazepoxide: 5-30 hours with active metabolites extending to 200+ hours).

B.2 Tapering Protocols

Standard taper (2025 guideline recommended): Reduce by 5-10% of the current dose every 2-4 weeks. Do not exceed 25% reduction in any 2-week period. The guideline emphasizes that this is a starting framework, and individualization is required. If withdrawal symptoms emerge, slow the taper or hold at the current dose until symptoms stabilize (Brunner et al., 2025).

Sample 10% taper schedule for a patient on alprazolam 2mg daily: Weeks 1-2: 2mg (baseline). Weeks 3-4: 1.8mg. Weeks 5-6: 1.6mg. Weeks 7-8: 1.4mg. Weeks 9-10: 1.25mg. Weeks 11-12: 1.1mg. Weeks 13-14: 1mg. Weeks 15-16: 0.875mg. Weeks 17-18: 0.75mg. Weeks 19-20: 0.625mg. Weeks 21-22: 0.5mg. Weeks 23-26: hyperbolic tapering at 5% or smaller reductions every 2-4 weeks. Total estimated duration: 6-9 months. This schedule illustrates why benzodiazepine tapering is a longitudinal clinical commitment, not a one-visit decision.

Hyperbolic tapering: The 2025 guideline recommends progressively smaller absolute dose reductions as the total dose decreases. This reflects the non-linear relationship between benzodiazepine dose and GABA-A receptor occupancy. Cutting from 2mg to 1.5mg reduces receptor occupancy by a modest percentage. Cutting from 0.5mg to 0mg eliminates a far larger percentage of remaining receptor occupancy. Clinically, this means the final 25% of the taper is often the most difficult and should proceed most slowly (Brunner et al., 2025).

Conversion to long-acting agent before taper: For patients on short-acting benzodiazepines (alprazolam, lorazepam) who experience significant interdose withdrawal, converting to a longer-acting equivalent (diazepam or clonazepam) before initiating the taper can smooth the withdrawal curve. Convert using the equivalency table (section B.1), divide the diazepam equivalent into 2-3 daily doses, stabilize for 1-2 weeks, then begin the taper protocol.

B.3 Adjunctive Support During Taper

Concurrent treatment for the condition that originally prompted benzodiazepine prescribing should be optimized before or during the taper. SSRI/SNRI for underlying anxiety disorder (section 7.1). CBT-I for insomnia (section 12.1). Hydroxyzine (25-50mg as needed) for breakthrough anxiety. Gabapentin (300-600mg at bedtime) for sleep support and anxiety. The 2025 guideline explicitly recommends offering patients adjunctive psychosocial interventions, particularly CBT, to support successful tapering (Brunner et al., 2025).

Appendix C: FDA Black Box Warning Reference

Black box warnings represent the FDA's highest level of safety alert. They signal risks that are life-threatening, require specific monitoring, or demand prescriber awareness to prevent serious harm. This appendix catalogs the black box warnings most relevant to psychiatric prescribing. The [BBW] icon used throughout this book references these warnings. Every prescriber should be familiar with the content of these warnings before prescribing the associated medications.

C.1 Antidepressant Warnings

All antidepressants (SSRIs, SNRIs, TCAs, MAOIs, bupropion, mirtazapine, trazodone, and others): Increased risk of suicidal thinking and behavior in children, adolescents, and young adults (under 25) during initial treatment (typically the first 1-2 months) or dose changes. Clinical monitoring is required: weekly for the first 4 weeks, biweekly for weeks 5-8, and at 12 weeks. This warning does not apply to patients over 25, for whom antidepressant treatment is associated with reduced suicidality. The warning should not deter appropriate antidepressant treatment in youth, as untreated depression carries a far higher suicide risk than treatment-emergent suicidal ideation (Hammad et al., 2006).

C.2 Antipsychotic Warnings

All antipsychotics (typical and atypical): Increased mortality in elderly patients with dementia-related psychosis. Causes of death were predominantly cardiovascular (heart failure, sudden death) or infectious (pneumonia). Antipsychotics are not FDA-approved for the treatment of dementia-related psychosis (with the exception of brexpiprazole for Alzheimer's agitation, and pimavanserin for

Parkinson's disease psychosis). This warning applies to both first-generation and second-generation agents. Off-label use in elderly dementia patients should be time-limited, regularly reassessed, and documented with informed consent (Stahl, 2021).

Clozapine: Severe neutropenia (formerly monitored through the Clozapine REMS, eliminated in 2025). Risk of potentially fatal agranulocytosis at a rate of approximately 0.38%. ANC monitoring is clinically required even after REMS elimination. Additional black box warnings for clozapine include: seizures (dose-related, approximately 5% at doses above 600mg), myocarditis and cardiomyopathy, and orthostatic hypotension with respiratory and cardiac arrest (particularly during initial titration).

C.3 Mood Stabilizer Warnings

Valproate (all formulations): Hepatotoxicity (potentially fatal, highest risk in children under 2, especially with mitochondrial disorders). Teratogenicity (neural tube defects, neurodevelopmental effects). Pancreatitis (rare but potentially life-threatening). These warnings make valproate contraindicated as first-line treatment in women of reproductive age.

Carbamazepine: Stevens-Johnson syndrome and toxic epidermal necrolysis, particularly in patients with HLA-B*1502 allele (highest prevalence in Southeast Asian populations). HLA testing is recommended before prescribing. Aplastic anemia and agranulocytosis (rare).

Lamotrigine: Serious skin reactions including Stevens-Johnson syndrome and toxic epidermal necrolysis. Risk is highest during the first 8 weeks of treatment and is increased by exceeding recommended titration schedules or by concurrent valproate use. The risk is managed through strict adherence to the slow titration protocol (Stahl, 2021).

Lithium: Lithium toxicity can occur at doses close to therapeutic levels. Toxicity produces irreversible neurological damage and can be fatal. Close monitoring of lithium levels, renal function, and drug interactions is required throughout treatment (section 22.4 for toxicity management).

C.4 Controlled Substance Warnings

All benzodiazepines and opioid combinations: Concurrent use of benzodiazepines and opioids increases the risk of respiratory depression, profound sedation, coma, and death. This boxed warning was added in 2016 and applies to all benzodiazepine prescriptions. Providers should limit concurrent prescribing, consider alternative treatments, and prescribe naloxone when the combination is unavoidable.

Z-drugs (zolpidem, zaleplon, eszopiclone): Complex sleep behaviors including sleep-walking, sleep-driving, and sleep-eating that can result in serious injury or death. These behaviors can occur after the first dose and at the lowest doses. Discontinue immediately if a patient reports complex sleep behaviors.

Stimulants (amphetamine and methylphenidate formulations): Potential for abuse and dependence. Serious cardiovascular adverse events including sudden death in patients with pre-existing structural cardiac abnormalities or other serious heart problems. Assess cardiovascular risk before prescribing (Stahl, 2021).

C.5 Other Relevant Warnings

Esketamine (Spravato): Sedation, dissociation, respiratory depression, and abuse potential. REMS requires administration in a certified healthcare setting with at least 2-hour observation. Patients cannot drive on the day of treatment.

Buprenorphine (all formulations): Risk of respiratory depression, particularly when combined with benzodiazepines, CNS depressants, or other opioids. Risk of neonatal opioid withdrawal syndrome. The boxed warning should not deter buprenorphine prescribing for OUD, as the mortality benefit of MOUD substantially outweighs these risks.

Nefazodone: Hepatic failure (removed from most markets but still available as generic). This is largely a historical note, as nefazodone is rarely prescribed.

Appendix D: New Medications 2024 to 2025

The pace of psychiatric drug development has accelerated in the 2024-2025 period, with novel mechanisms of action, expanded indications for existing agents, regulatory changes that improve access, and new formulations that address practical clinical barriers. This appendix consolidates these developments as a quick reference. Each entry includes the clinical positioning that helps you decide when to consider the new option versus established treatments.

D.1 Novel Approvals

Cobenfy (xanomeline/trospium): Approved September 2024 for schizophrenia. First antipsychotic with a non-dopaminergic mechanism. Xanomeline is a muscarinic M1/M4 receptor agonist. Trospium is a peripheral muscarinic antagonist that does not cross the blood-brain barrier, included to mitigate peripheral cholinergic side effects (nausea, constipation, dyspepsia). Dosing: 50mg/20mg twice daily, titrated to 125mg/30mg twice daily. No black box warning. Favorable metabolic, EPS, and prolactin profile compared to dopamine-blocking antipsychotics. Clinical positioning: consider for patients with significant metabolic risk, EPS sensitivity, or hyperprolactinemia concerns requiring antipsychotic treatment (Kaul et al., 2024).

Esketamine (Spravato) monotherapy for TRD: Supplemental approval 2025. Previously approved only in conjunction with an oral antidepressant. Monotherapy approval allows initiation without adding a new daily oral antidepressant, which is relevant for patients with significant intolerance to oral antidepressants, high pill burden, or polypharmacy. The 84mg dose demonstrated effect sizes of 0.63 versus placebo. REMS, clinic-based administration, and 2-hour observation requirements remain unchanged (Daly et al., 2019).

Lumateperone (Caplyta) for adjunctive MDD: Expanded indication approved 2025. Previously approved for schizophrenia and bipolar I/II depression. Dosing for MDD augmentation: 42mg daily. Acts through serotonin, dopamine, and glutamate modulation. Favorable metabolic and movement disorder profile compared to other atypical antipsychotics used for MDD augmentation (aripiprazole, brexpiprazole, quetiapine XR). Clinical positioning: consider when standard MDD augmentation agents produce intolerable weight gain, akathisia, or metabolic effects (Durgam et al., 2024).

Cyclobenzaprine sublingual (Tonmya): Approved 2025 for fibromyalgia. Low-dose sublingual formulation that targets the sleep-pain cycle. Acts on serotonergic and noradrenergic pathways at doses below the muscle relaxant threshold, reducing central pain sensitization and improving sleep architecture. Clinical positioning: consider for fibromyalgia patients with prominent sleep disruption who have not responded adequately to duloxetine or pregabalin alone.

D.2 Expanded Indications

Iloperidone (Fanapt) for bipolar I disorder: FDA approval 2024 for manic and mixed episodes. Atypical antipsychotic with relatively favorable EPS profile but requires slow titration due to orthostatic hypotension risk (start 1mg twice daily, titrate over 7 days to target 6-12mg twice daily). CYP2D6 and CYP3A4 substrate. Clinical positioning: alternative for acute mania when other agents are contraindicated or poorly tolerated.

UZEDY (risperidone) for bipolar I maintenance: Expanded indication 2025. Extended-release subcutaneous injection (monthly administration). Provides long-acting risperidone without the deltoid/gluteal IM injection requirement of Risperdal Consta. Clinical positioning: bipolar I maintenance when adherence is a concern and the patient tolerates risperidone.

Erzofri (paliperidone palmitate): Approved 2024. Simplified single first-month injection for schizophrenia, eliminating the two-injection initiation sequence required by Invega Sustenna. Clinical positioning: reduces the logistical barrier to LAI initiation and may improve transition rates from oral to injectable antipsychotics.

D.3 Formulation and Access Changes

Onyda XR (clonidine extended-release oral suspension): Approved 2024 for ADHD in pediatric patients aged 6 and above. Liquid suspension formulation of the alpha-2 agonist already approved in tablet form (Kapvay). Clinical positioning: pediatric patients who cannot swallow tablets, patients requiring precise dose titration.

Ingrezza Sprinkle (valbenazine): Approved 2024. Sprinkle capsule formulation of the VMAT2 inhibitor for tardive dyskinesia. Capsule can be opened and contents sprinkled on food. Clinical positioning: patients with TD who have dysphagia or difficulty swallowing capsules.

Zunveyl (benzgalantamine): Approved 2024 for Alzheimer's disease. Delayed-release formulation of a galantamine precursor designed to reduce the GI side effects that limit cholinesterase inhibitor tolerability. Clinical positioning: Alzheimer's patients who discontinued galantamine or other ChEIs due to nausea and vomiting.

D.4 Regulatory and Guideline Changes

Clozapine REMS elimination (June 2025): The FDA eliminated the Clozapine Risk Evaluation and Mitigation Strategy program. Prescribers and pharmacies are no longer required to enroll patients in a centralized database or obtain dispense authorization before each fill. The risk of severe neutropenia persists, and ANC monitoring remains clinically required (section 10.3). Clinical impact: removes administrative barriers that delayed clozapine initiation and contributed to underutilization of the only evidence-based treatment for treatment-resistant schizophrenia.

2025 FDA class-wide ER stimulant label update: Added a clearer limitation-of-use signal for extended-release amphetamine and methylphenidate formulations in children under 6 years. Reflects higher plasma exposure and higher rates of adverse effects (including clinically significant weight loss) in this age group compared to older children at the same dosage. Clinical impact: reinforces that behavioral interventions should be attempted first in preschool-aged children.

2025 Joint Clinical Practice Guideline on Benzodiazepine Tapering: Developed by 10 medical societies led by ASAM. Key recommendations: risk-benefit reassessment every 3 months, taper pace of 5-10% every 2-4 weeks, hyperbolic tapering at lower doses, adjunctive CBT support, and the distinction between physical dependence (expected with chronic use) and substance use disorder. See section 7.4 for full clinical application.

2025 APA Delirium Guidelines: Recommend against antipsychotics for delirium prevention or routine treatment. Reserve antipsychotics for severe agitation or distress posing safety risks, only after nonpharmacologic strategies and reversible contributors are addressed. Recommend dexmedetomidine over other sedating agents for surgical delirium prevention. See section 20.4 for clinical application.

Lumipulse blood test for Alzheimer's diagnosis (2025): First FDA-cleared blood test to aid Alzheimer's diagnosis in cognitively impaired adults. May simplify the diagnostic pathway for anti-amyloid therapy eligibility by reducing dependence on amyloid PET imaging.

D.5 Pipeline to Watch

Milsaperidone (Bysanti): NDA submitted for bipolar I disorder and schizophrenia. Active metabolite of iloperidone targeting HTR2 and DRD2 receptors. Potential US availability 2026. **MM120 (lysergide)**: Phase 3 study initiated for MDD, results expected second half 2026. Psychedelic-assisted therapy model. **Ecopipam**: Novel D1 receptor antagonist for Tourette syndrome. Positive 12-month open-label extension data in pediatric patients (2025). First-in-class mechanism that avoids D2 blockade (Gilbert et al., 2018).

Appendix E: Pharmacogenomic Reference

This appendix consolidates the pharmacogenomic information referenced throughout the book into quick-lookup tables. Chapter 3.0 provides the clinical framework for ordering, interpreting, and applying pharmacogenomic results. This appendix provides the specific gene-drug-phenotype reference data.

E.1 CYP2D6 Clinical Reference

Key substrates (medications whose levels are affected by CYP2D6 status): aripiprazole, brexpiprazole, risperidone, haloperidol, perphenazine, iloperidone, fluoxetine, paroxetine, fluvoxamine, venlafaxine (conversion to active metabolite), nortriptyline, desipramine, amitriptyline, imipramine, atomoxetine, codeine (prodrug activation), tramadol (prodrug activation), dextromethorphan.

Potent inhibitors (medications that functionally shift CYP2D6 normal metabolizers toward poor metabolizer status): fluoxetine, paroxetine, bupropion, quinidine. **Moderate inhibitors**: duloxetine, sertraline (at higher doses), terbinafine.

CPIC dose adjustment guidance: CYP2D6 poor metabolizers receiving aripiprazole should have the dose reduced by approximately 50%. CYP2D6 poor metabolizers receiving TCAs (nortriptyline, desipramine, amitriptyline) should start at 25% of normal dose with therapeutic drug monitoring. CYP2D6 ultra-rapid metabolizers on codeine should avoid codeine entirely (excessive morphine production). CYP2D6 ultra-rapid metabolizers on TCAs may require higher doses guided by drug levels (Hicks et al., 2015; Hicks et al., 2017).

Phenoconversion alert: A patient with normal CYP2D6 genotype who is also taking fluoxetine (a potent 2D6 inhibitor) is functionally a poor metabolizer. Always assess the current medication list alongside genetic results (Mostafa et al., 2022).

E.2 CYP2C19 Clinical Reference

Key substrates: citalopram, escitalopram, sertraline (partial), diazepam, clobazam, phenytoin, proton pump inhibitors (omeprazole, esomeprazole, lansoprazole, pantoprazole). **Potent inhibitors**: fluvoxamine. **Moderate inhibitors**: fluoxetine, omeprazole.

CPIC dose adjustment guidance: CYP2C19 poor metabolizers receiving citalopram should have a 50% dose reduction (maximum 20mg). CYP2C19 poor metabolizers receiving escitalopram should consider a 50% dose reduction. CYP2C19 ultra-rapid metabolizers receiving citalopram or escitalopram may need higher doses or an alternative agent, as standard doses may produce subtherapeutic levels. CYP2C19 poor metabolizers receiving clobazam (for seizure disorders) require significant dose reduction (Hicks et al., 2015).

E.3 CYP3A4 Clinical Reference

Key substrates: quetiapine, lurasidone, buspirone, alprazolam, midazolam, triazolam, carbamazepine (auto-inducer), pimozide, ziprasidone. **Potent inhibitors**: ketoconazole, itraconazole, clarithromycin, ritonavir, nefazodone, grapefruit juice. **Potent inducers**: carbamazepine, phenytoin, phenobarbital, rifampin, St. John's Wort.

Clinical implications: Adding a potent CYP3A4 inhibitor to a patient on quetiapine or lurasidone can dramatically increase antipsychotic levels. Adding a potent inducer (carbamazepine) can reduce levels to subtherapeutic range. Lurasidone labeling contraindicates concurrent use with potent CYP3A4 inhibitors or inducers (Stahl, 2021).

E.4 CYP1A2 Clinical Reference

Key substrates: clozapine, olanzapine, duloxetine, fluvoxamine, theophylline, caffeine. **Inducers**: smoking (polycyclic aromatic hydrocarbons from combustion, not nicotine), charbroiled foods. **Potent inhibitor**: fluvoxamine.

Clinical implications: Smoking cessation in a patient on clozapine will raise clozapine levels 50-70% over 2-4 weeks. Proactively reduce clozapine dose by 25-50% when a patient quits smoking. Nicotine replacement therapy (patches, gum, lozenges) does not induce CYP1A2. Fluvoxamine should generally be avoided in patients on clozapine or olanzapine due to the potent CYP1A2 inhibition that raises substrate levels substantially (Stahl, 2021).

E.5 HLA Screening Reference

*_HLA-B_1502**: Test before prescribing carbamazepine or oxcarbazepine to patients of Southeast Asian ancestry (Han Chinese, Filipino, Malaysian, South Asian Indian, Thai). Positive result is a contraindication to carbamazepine use. Prevalence: approximately 5-15% in Southeast Asian populations, less than 1% in European and African populations (Leckband et al., 2013).

*_HLA-A_3101**: Test before prescribing carbamazepine to patients of European, Japanese, or Korean ancestry. Positive result indicates increased risk of carbamazepine-induced hypersensitivity reactions (SJS/TEN and DRESS syndrome). Prevalence: approximately 2-5% in European populations, 9-10% in Japanese populations. Clinical decision: positive result warrants use of an alternative mood stabilizer or anticonvulsant (Leckband et al., 2013).

E.6 CPIC Guideline Summary

As of 2024, CPIC and DPWG have collectively published pharmacogenomic prescribing guidelines for the following psychiatric medications:

Antidepressants (14 medications): amitriptyline, citalopram, clomipramine, desipramine, doxepin, escitalopram, fluvoxamine, imipramine, nortriptyline, paroxetine, sertraline, trimipramine, venlafaxine, vortioxetine. Guidelines primarily address CYP2D6 and CYP2C19 genotype-based dosing.

Antipsychotics (7 medications): aripiprazole, brexpiprazole, haloperidol, pimozide, risperidone, thioridazine, zuclopenthixol. Guidelines primarily address CYP2D6 genotype-based dosing.

Anticonvulsant/Mood stabilizers (3 medications): carbamazepine, oxcarbazepine, phenytoin. Guidelines address HLA genotype-based prescribing decisions and CYP2C9/CYP2C19 for phenytoin.

ADHD (1 medication): atomoxetine. Guideline addresses CYP2D6 genotype-based dosing (Brown et al., 2019; Hicks et al., 2015; Hicks et al., 2017; Leckband et al., 2013).

Appendix F: Resources and References

This appendix compiles the clinical resources, databases, practice guidelines, and professional tools referenced throughout the book. Resources are organized by category for rapid clinical access. All URLs were verified as of publication date. Digital resources change frequently; if a link is no longer active, search the organization name directly.

F.1 Practice Guidelines Cited

American Psychiatric Association (APA): Practice guideline for the treatment of patients with major depressive disorder (3rd ed., 2010). Practice guideline for bipolar disorder (under revision). Practice guidelines for the prevention and management of delirium (2025). Accessed at psychiatry.org/psychiatrists/practice/clinical-practice-guidelines.

VA/DoD Clinical Practice Guidelines: Management of major depressive disorder (2022). Management of posttraumatic stress disorder and acute stress reaction (2017). Assessment and management of patients at risk for suicide (2019). Accessed at healthquality.va.gov.

Canadian Network for Mood and Anxiety Treatments (CANMAT): CANMAT and ISBD 2018 guidelines for the management of patients with bipolar disorder (Yatham et al., 2018). CANMAT 2023 guidelines for the management of adults with major depressive disorder (under revision). Accessed at canmat.org.

National Institute for Health and Care Excellence (NICE): Depression in adults: treatment and management (2022 update). Generalized anxiety disorder and panic disorder in adults (2019 update). Bipolar disorder: assessment and management (2023 update). Accessed at nice.org.uk.

American Society of Addiction Medicine (ASAM): Joint clinical practice guideline on benzodiazepine tapering (2025). ASAM criteria for the treatment of addictive, substance-related, and co-occurring conditions. Accessed at asam.org.

American College of Obstetricians and Gynecologists (ACOG): Clinical practice guideline number 5: Treatment and management of mental health conditions during pregnancy and postpartum (2023). Accessed at acog.org.

Clinical Pharmacogenetics Implementation Consortium (CPIC): Peer-reviewed, freely available pharmacogenomic prescribing guidelines for antidepressants, antipsychotics, mood stabilizers, and atomoxetine. Accessed at cpicpgx.org/guidelines.

F.2 Clinical Decision Support Tools

LactMed: National Library of Medicine database on drugs and lactation. Free, regularly updated, evidence-based. Accessed at ncbi.nlm.nih.gov/books/NBK501922.

InfantRisk Center: Provider consultation service from Texas Tech University Health Sciences Center. Phone consultations available for prescribers making lactation safety decisions. Accessed at infantrisk.com.

MotherToBaby: Patient-facing fact sheets on medication safety during pregnancy and breastfeeding, maintained by the Organization of Teratology Information Specialists. Accessed at mothertobaby.org.

Reprotox: Subscription-based database highlighting medication effects during pregnancy, breastfeeding, and development. Accessed at reprotox.org.

PharmGKB (Pharmacogenomics Knowledge Base): Curates pharmacogenomic data and CPIC guideline information. Free access. Accessed at pharmgkb.org.

Lexicomp and Micromedex: Subscription-based drug interaction databases used in clinical settings. Available through most hospital and health system pharmacies.

F.3 Rating Scale Resources

PHQ-9: Freely available. No copyright restrictions on clinical use. Available at phqscreeners.com.

GAD-7: Freely available. Developed by Drs. Spitzer, Kroenke, and Williams. Available at phqscreeners.com.

MDQ (Mood Disorder Questionnaire): Freely available for clinical use. Published by Hirschfeld et al. (2000).

Columbia Suicide Severity Rating Scale (C-SSRS): Freely available. Multiple versions for clinical settings. Accessed at cssrs.columbia.edu.

PCL-5 (PTSD Checklist for DSM-5): Freely available from the National Center for PTSD. Accessed at ptsd.va.gov.

AUDIT-C: Freely available alcohol screening tool. 3-item version of the full AUDIT. Widely reproduced in clinical guidelines.

ASRS (Adult ADHD Self-Report Scale): Freely available 6-item screener and 18-item symptom checklist. Developed by the World Health Organization. Accessed at hcp.med.harvard.edu/ncs/asrs.php.

F.4 Professional Development Resources

Psychopharmacology Institute: CME-accredited psychopharmacology education. Annual reviews of FDA approvals and practice guideline changes. Accessed at psychopharmacologyinstitute.com.

PsychDB: Free, open-access clinical psychiatry database with guideline summaries, prescribing algorithms, and teaching resources. Accessed at psychdb.com.

Harvard South Shore Psychopharmacology Algorithm Project: Published evidence-based prescribing algorithms for depression, bipolar disorder, PTSD, GAD, schizophrenia, and other conditions. Available through published journal articles and at psychopharm.mobi.

AAPP (American Association of Psychiatric Pharmacists): Professional organization for psychiatric pharmacy. Guidelines, education, and consultation resources. Accessed at aapp.org.

F.5 Regulatory and Monitoring Resources

PDMP (Prescription Drug Monitoring Program): State-specific databases for tracking controlled substance prescriptions. Access points vary by state. The NABP PMP InterConnect system enables interstate data sharing. Accessed through individual state pharmacy board websites.

FDA MedWatch: Adverse event reporting and drug safety information. Prescribers can report suspected adverse events. Accessed at fda.gov/safety/medwatch-fda-safety-information-and-adverse-event-reporting-program.

DEA Diversion Control Division: Registration requirements, controlled substance schedules, and prescribing regulations. Accessed at deadiversion.usdoj.gov.

Perinatal Psychiatry Access Programs: State-based programs connecting clinicians with perinatal psychiatrists and resource specialists. National coverage through Postpartum Support International's Perinatal Psychiatric Consult Line. Directory accessed at postpartum.net and lifeline4moms.org.

988 Suicide and Crisis Lifeline: Available 24/7 by phone, chat, or text for individuals in crisis. Formerly the National Suicide Prevention Lifeline. Prescribers can provide this resource to patients during medication visits when suicide risk is identified.

F.6 Key Textbook References

Sadock, B. J., Sadock, V. A., & Ruiz, P. (2015). *Kaplan and Sadock's synopsis of psychiatry* (11th ed.). Wolters Kluwer.

Schatzberg, A. F., & Nemeroff, C. B. (2017). *The American Psychiatric Association Publishing textbook of psychopharmacology* (5th ed.). American Psychiatric Association Publishing.

Stahl, S. M. (2021). *Stahl's essential psychopharmacology: Neuroscientific basis and practical applications* (5th ed.). Cambridge University Press.

Stahl, S. M. (2024). *Stahl's essential psychopharmacology: Prescriber's guide* (8th ed.). Cambridge University Press.

Taylor, D., Barnes, T. R. E., & Young, A. H. (2021). *The Maudsley prescribing guidelines in psychiatry* (14th ed.). Wiley-Blackwell.

References

American College of Obstetricians and Gynecologists. (2023). Clinical practice guideline number 5: Treatment and management of mental health conditions during pregnancy and postpartum. *Obstetrics & Gynecology, 141*(6), 1262–1288.

American Diabetes Association, American Psychiatric Association, American Association of Clinical Endocrinologists, & North American Association for the Study of Obesity. (2004). Consensus development conference on antipsychotic drugs and obesity and diabetes. *Diabetes Care, 27*(2), 596–601.

American Geriatrics Society 2023 Beers Criteria® Update Expert Panel. (2023). American Geriatrics Society 2023 updated AGS Beers Criteria® for potentially inappropriate medication use in older adults. *Journal of the American Geriatrics Society, 71*(7), 2052–2081.

American Psychiatric Association. (2009). *Practice guideline for the treatment of patients with panic disorder* (2nd ed.). American Psychiatric Association.

American Psychiatric Association. (2010). *Practice guideline for the treatment of patients with major depressive disorder* (3rd ed.). American Psychiatric Association.

American Psychiatric Association. (2022). *Diagnostic and statistical manual of mental disorders* (5th ed., text rev.). American Psychiatric Association Publishing.

American Psychiatric Association. (2025). *Practice guideline for the prevention and treatment of delirium*. American Psychiatric Association.

Attia, E., Steinglass, J. E., Walsh, B. T., Wang, Y., Wu, P., Schreyer, C., Wildes, J., Yilmaz, Z., Guarda, A. S., Kaplan, A. S., & Marcus, M. D. (2019). Olanzapine versus placebo in adult outpatients with anorexia nervosa: A randomized clinical trial. *American Journal of Psychiatry, 176*(6), 449–456.

Bajor, L. A., Balsara, C., & Osser, D. N. (2025). Posttraumatic stress disorder psychopharmacology algorithm update—2024–2025. *Psychiatry and Clinical Psychopharmacology, 35*(Suppl. 1), S135–S140.

Bandelow, B., Michaelis, S., & Wedekind, D. (2017). Treatment of anxiety disorders. *Dialogues in Clinical Neuroscience, 19*(2), 93–107.

Beach, S. R., Celano, C. M., Noseworthy, P. A., Januzzi, J. L., & Huffman, J. C. (2013). QTc prolongation, torsades de pointes, and psychotropic medications. *Psychosomatics, 54*(1), 1–13.

Blier, P. (2014). Rational site-directed pharmacotherapy for major depressive disorder. *International Journal of Neuropsychopharmacology, 17*(7), 997–1008.

Bloch, M. H., Landeros-Weisenberger, A., Kelmendi, B., Coric, V., Bracken, M. B., & Leckman, J. F. (2006). A systematic review: Antipsychotic augmentation with treatment refractory obsessive-compulsive disorder. *Molecular Psychiatry, 11*(7), 622–632.

Bousman, C. A., Bengesser, S. A., Aitchison, K. J., Amare, A. T., Aschauer, H., Baune, B. T., Batra, R., Bishop, J. R., Burmeister, M., Chaumette, B., Chen, L. S., Cordeiro, Q., Dalton, R., DeLisi, L. E., Eriksson, L. I., Frye, M. A., Fullerton, J. M., Gennarelli, M., Goes, F. S., ... Mueller, D. J. (2021). Review and consensus on pharmacogenomic testing in psychiatry. *Pharmacopsychiatry, 54*(1), 5–17.

Bovin, M. J., Marx, B. P., Weathers, F. W., Gallagher, M. W., Rodriguez, P., Schnurr, P. P., & Keane, T. M. (2016). Psychometric properties of the PTSD Checklist for Diagnostic and Statistical Manual of Mental Disorders, Fifth Edition (PCL-5) in veterans. *Psychological Assessment, 28*(11), 1379–1391.

Boyer, E. W., & Shannon, M. (2005). The serotonin syndrome. *New England Journal of Medicine, 352*(11), 1112–1120.

Brown, J. T., Bishop, J. R., Sangkuhl, K., Nurmi, E. L., Mueller, D. J., Dinh, J. C., Gaedigk, A., Klein, T. E., Caudle, K. E., McCracken, J. T., de Leon, J., & Leeder, J. S. (2019). Clinical Pharmacogenetics Implementation Consortium guideline for cytochrome P450

(CYP)2D6 genotype and atomoxetine therapy. *Clinical Pharmacology & Therapeutics, 106*(1), 94–102.

Brunner, E., Chen, C. A., Engel, L., Fareed, N., Gelenberg, A. J., Maust, D. T., Nunes, E. V., Oesterle, T. S., Reidenberg, M. M., Tirado, C. F., VandenBerg, A., Yager, J., & Zgierska, A. E. (2025). Joint clinical practice guideline on benzodiazepine tapering: Considerations when risks outweigh benefits. *Journal of General Internal Medicine, 40*(12), 2814–2859.

Calabrese, J. R., Keck, P. E., Macfadden, W., Minkwitz, M., Ketter, T. A., Weisler, R. H., Cutler, A. J., McCoy, R., Wilson, E., & Mullen, J. (2005). A randomized, double-blind, placebo-controlled trial of quetiapine in the treatment of bipolar I or II depression. *American Journal of Psychiatry, 162*(7), 1351–1360.

Celada, P., Puig, M. V., & Artigas, F. (2013). Serotonin modulation of cortical neurons and networks. *Frontiers in Integrative Neuroscience, 7*, Article 25.

Cipriani, A., Furukawa, T. A., Salanti, G., Chaimani, A., Atkinson, L. Z., Ogawa, Y., Leucht, S., Ruhe, H. G., Turner, E. H., Higgins, J. P. T., Egger, M., Takeshima, N., Hayasaka, Y., Imai, H., Shinohara, K., Tajika, A., Ioannidis, J. P. A., & Geddes, J. R. (2018). Comparative efficacy and acceptability of 21 antidepressant drugs for the acute treatment of adults with major depressive disorder: A systematic review and network meta-analysis. *The Lancet, 391*(10128), 1357–1366.

Cipriani, A., Hawton, K., Stockton, S., & Geddes, J. R. (2013). Lithium in the prevention of suicide in mood disorders: Updated systematic review and meta-analysis. *BMJ, 346*, f3646.

Correll, C. U., Citrome, L., Haddad, P. M., Lauriello, J., Olfson, M., Calloway, S. M., & Kane, J. M. (2016). The use of long-acting injectable antipsychotics in schizophrenia: Evaluating the evidence. *Journal of Clinical Psychiatry, 77*(Suppl. 3), 1–24.

Correll, C. U., Manu, P., Olshanskiy, V., Napolitano, B., Kane, J. M., & Malhotra, A. K. (2009). Cardiometabolic risk of second-generation antipsychotic medications during first-time use in children and adolescents. *JAMA, 302*(16), 1765–1773.

Correll, C. U., Robinson, D. G., Schooler, N. R., Brunette, M. F., Mueser, K. T., Rosenheck, R. A., Marcy, P., Addington, J., Estroff, S. E., Robinson, J., Penn, D. L., Azrin, S., Goldstein, A., Severe, J., Heinssen, R., & Kane, J. M. (2014). Cardiometabolic risk in patients with first-episode schizophrenia spectrum disorders: Baseline results from the RAISE-ETP study. *JAMA Psychiatry, 71*(12), 1350–1363.

Corrigan, P. W., Druss, B. G., & Perlick, D. A. (2014). The impact of mental illness stigma on seeking and participating in mental health care. *Psychological Science in the Public Interest, 15*(2), 37–70.

Daly, E. J., Singh, J. B., Fedgchin, M., Cooper, K., Lim, P., Shelton, R. C., Thase, M. E., Winokur, A., Van Nueten, L., Manji, H., & Drevets, W. C. (2018). Efficacy and safety of intranasal esketamine adjunctive to oral antidepressant therapy in treatment-resistant depression: A randomized clinical trial. *JAMA Psychiatry, 75*(2), 139–148.

Decker, B. S., Goldfarb, D. S., Dargan, P. I., Friesen, M., Gosselin, S., Hoffman, R. S., Lavergne, V., Nolin, T. D., & Ghannoum, M. (2015). Extracorporeal treatment for lithium poisoning: Systematic review and recommendations from the EXTRIP workgroup. *Clinical Journal of the American Society of Nephrology, 10*(5), 875–887.

Deegan, P. E., & Drake, R. E. (2006). Shared decision making and medication management in the recovery process. *Psychiatric Services, 57*(11), 1636–1639.

Deligiannidis, K. M., Meltzer-Brody, S., Maximos, B., Peeper, E. Q., Freeman, M., Lasser, R., Bullock, A., Kotecha, M., Li, S., Forrestal, F., Rana, N., Garcia, M., Leclair, B., & Bhatt, D. K. (2023). Zuranolone for the treatment of postpartum depression. *American Journal of Psychiatry, 180*(9), 668–675.

Durgam, S., Earley, W., Kozauer, S. G., Chen, C., Lakkis, H., Edwards, J. B., & Stahl, S. (2024). Lumateperone as adjunctive therapy in patients with major depressive disorder: Results from a randomized, double-blind, phase 3 trial. *Neuroscience Applied, 3*, Article 104586.

Faraone, S. V. (2018). The pharmacology of amphetamine and methylphenidate: Relevance to the neurobiology of attention-deficit/hyperactivity disorder and other psychiatric comorbidities. *Neuroscience & Biobehavioral Reviews, 87*, 255–270.

Friedman, M. J., Keane, T. M., & Resick, P. A. (Eds.). (2014). *Handbook of PTSD: Science and practice* (2nd ed.). Guilford Press.

Gilbert, D. L., Budman, C. L., Singer, H. S., Kurlan, R., & Chipkin, R. E. (2018). A D1 receptor antagonist, ecopipam, for treatment of tics in Tourette syndrome. *Clinical Neuropharmacology, 41*(1), 2–8.

Glassman, A. H., O'Connor, C. M., Califf, R. M., Swedberg, K., Schwartz, P., Bigger, J. T., Krishnan, K. R. R., van Zyl, L. T., Swenson, J. R., Finkel, M. S., Landau, C., Shapiro, P. A., Pepine, C. J., Mardekian, J., Harrison, W. M., Barton, D., & McIvor, M. (2002). Sertraline treatment of major depression in patients with acute MI or unstable angina. *JAMA, 288*(6), 701–709.

Grant, J. E., Odlaug, B. L., & Kim, S. W. (2009). N-acetylcysteine, a glutamate modulator, in the treatment of trichotillomania: A double-blind, placebo-controlled study. *Archives of General Psychiatry, 66*(7), 756–763.

Gray, K. M., Carpenter, M. J., Baker, N. L., DeSantis, S. M., Kryway, E., Hartwell, K. J., McRae-Clark, A. L., & Brady, K. T. (2012). A double-blind randomized controlled trial of N-acetylcysteine in cannabis-dependent adolescents. *American Journal of Psychiatry, 169*(8), 805–812.

Greden, J. F., Parikh, S. V., Rothschild, A. J., Thase, M. E., Dunlop, B. W., DeBattista, C., Conway, C. R., Forester, B. P., Mondimore, F. M., Shelton, R. C., Trivedi, M. H., & Keller, M. B. (2019). Impact of pharmacogenomics on clinical outcomes in major depressive disorder in the GUIDED trial. *Journal of Psychiatric Research, 111*, 59–67.

Hammad, T. A., Laughren, T., & Racoosin, J. (2006). Suicidality in pediatric patients treated with antidepressant drugs. *Archives of General Psychiatry, 63*(3), 332–339.

Herring, W. J., Connor, K. M., Ivgy-May, N., Snyder, E., Liu, K., Snavely, D. B., Krystal, A. D., Walsh, J. K., Benca, R. M., Rosenberg, R., Sangal, R. B., Budd, K., Hutzelmann, J., Leibensperger, H., Froman, S., Lines, C., Roth, T., & Michelson, D. (2016). Suvorexant in patients with insomnia: Results from two 3-month randomized controlled clinical trials. *Biological Psychiatry, 79*(2), 136–148.

Hicks, J. K., Bishop, J. R., Sangkuhl, K., Müller, D. J., Ji, Y., Leckband, S. G., Leeder, J. S., Graham, R. L., Chiulli, D. L., LLerena, A., Skaar, T. C., Scott, S. A., Stingl, J. C., Klein, T. E., Caudle, K. E., & Gaedigk, A. (2015). Clinical Pharmacogenetics Implementation Consortium (CPIC) guideline for CYP2D6 and CYP2C19 genotypes and dosing of selective serotonin reuptake inhibitors. *Clinical Pharmacology & Therapeutics, 98*(2), 127–134.

Hicks, J. K., Sangkuhl, K., Swen, J. J., Ellingrod, V. L., Müller, D. J., Shimoda, K., Bishop, J. R., Kharasch, E. D., Skaar, T. C., Gaedigk, A., Dunnenberger, H. M., Klein, T. E., Caudle, K. E., & Stingl, J. C. (2017). Clinical Pharmacogenetics Implementation Consortium guideline for CYP2D6 and CYP2C19 genotypes and dosing of tricyclic antidepressants: 2016 update. *Clinical Pharmacology & Therapeutics, 102*(1), 37–44.

Hiemke, C., & Hartter, S. (2000). Pharmacokinetics of selective serotonin reuptake inhibitors. *Pharmacology & Therapeutics, 85*(1), 11–28.

Hirschfeld, R. M. A., Williams, J. B. W., Spitzer, R. L., Calabrese, J. R., Flynn, L., Keck, P. E., Lewis, L., McElroy, S. L., Post, R. M., Rapport, D. J., Russell, J. M., Sachs, G. S., & Zajecka, J. (2000). Development and validation of a screening instrument for bipolar spectrum disorder: The Mood Disorder Questionnaire. *American Journal of Psychiatry, 157*(11), 1873–1875.

Horowitz, M. A., & Taylor, D. (2019). Tapering of SSRI treatment to mitigate withdrawal symptoms. *The Lancet Psychiatry, 6*(6), 538–546.

Howes, O. D., & Kapur, S. (2009). The dopamine hypothesis of schizophrenia: Version III—The final common pathway. *Schizophrenia Bulletin, 35*(3), 549–562.

Huybrechts, K. F., Palmsten, K., Avorn, J., Cohen, L. S., Holmes, L. B., Franklin, J. M., Mogun, H., Levin, R., Kowal, M., Setoguchi, S., & Hernández-Díaz, S. (2014). Antidepressant use in pregnancy and the risk of cardiac defects. *New England Journal of Medicine, 370*(25), 2397–2407.

Iosifescu, D. V., Jones, A., O'Gorman, C., Streicher, C., Felber, H., Kotecha, M., Nandi, P., Kott, A., & Daly, E. J. (2022). Efficacy and safety of AXS-05 (dextromethorphan-bupropion) in patients with major depressive disorder: A phase 3 randomized clinical trial (GEMINI). *Journal of Clinical Psychiatry, 83*(4), Article 21m14345.

Ipser, J. C., Kariuki, C. M., & Stein, D. J. (2008). Pharmacotherapy for social anxiety disorder: A systematic review. *Expert Review of Neurotherapeutics, 8*(2), 235–257.

Jonas, D. E., Amick, H. R., Feltner, C., Bobashev, G., Thomas, K., Wines, R., Kim, M. M., Shanahan, E., Gass, C. E., Rowe, C. J., & Garbutt, J. C. (2014). Pharmacotherapy for adults with alcohol use disorders in outpatient settings: A systematic review and meta-analysis. *JAMA, 311*(18), 1889–1900.

Kapur, S., Zipursky, R., Jones, C., Remington, G., & Houle, S. (2000). Relationship between dopamine D2 occupancy, clinical response, and side effects: A double-blind PET study of first-episode schizophrenia. *American Journal of Psychiatry, 157*(4), 514–520.

Kaul, I., Sawchak, S., Correll, C. U., Kakar, R., Breier, A., Zhu, H., Miller, A. C., Paul, S. M., & Brannan, S. K. (2024). Efficacy and safety of the muscarinic receptor agonist KarXT (xanomeline-trospium) in schizophrenia (EMERGENT-2): Results from a randomised, double-blind, placebo-controlled, flexible-dose phase 3 trial. *The Lancet, 403*(10422), 160–170.

Kellner, C. H., Greenberg, R. M., Murrough, J. W., Bryson, E. O., Briggs, M. C., & Pasculli, R. M. (2012). ECT in treatment-resistant depression. *American Journal of Psychiatry, 169*(12), 1238–1244.

Kessler, R. C., Adler, L., Ames, M., Demler, O., Faraone, S., Hiripi, E., Howes, M. J., Jin, R., Secnik, K., Spencer, T., Ustun, T. B., & Walters, E. E. (2005). The World Health Organization Adult ADHD Self-Report Scale (ASRS): A short screening scale for use in the general population. *Psychological Medicine, 35*(2), 245–256.

Kooij, J. J. S., Bijlenga, D., Salerno, L., Jaeschke, R., Bitter, I., Balázs, J., Thome, J., Dom, G., Kasper, S., Nunes-Filipe, C., Stes, S., Mohr, P., Grevet, E. H., Oliveira, C., Stringaris, A., Bergink, V., Asherson, P., Dias, G., Kiss, E., ... Adamou, M. (2019). Updated European consensus statement on diagnosis and treatment of adult ADHD. *European Psychiatry, 56*, 14–34.

Kroenke, K., Spitzer, R. L., & Williams, J. B. W. (2001). The PHQ-9: Validity of a brief depression severity measure. *Journal of General Internal Medicine, 16*(9), 606–613.

Lavretsky, H., Reinlieb, M., St. Cyr, N., Siddarth, P., Ercoli, L. M., & Senturk, D. (2015). Citalopram, methylphenidate, or their combination in geriatric depression: A randomized, double-blind, placebo-controlled trial. *American Journal of Psychiatry, 172*(6), 561–569.

Leckband, S. G., Kelsoe, J. R., Dunnenberger, H. M., George, A. L., Tran, E., Berger, R., Müller, D. J., Whirl-Carrillo, M., Caudle, K. E., & Pirmohamed, M. (2013). Clinical Pharmacogenetics Implementation Consortium guidelines for HLA-B genotype and carbamazepine dosing. *Clinical Pharmacology & Therapeutics, 94*(3), 324–328.

Lieb, K., Völlm, B., Rücker, G., Timmer, A., & Stoffers, J. M. (2010). Pharmacotherapy for borderline personality disorder: Cochrane systematic review of randomised trials. *British Journal of Psychiatry, 196*(1), 4–12.

Malhi, G. S., Tanious, M., Das, P., Coulston, C. M., & Berk, M. (2013). Potential mechanisms of action of lithium in bipolar disorder: Current understanding. *CNS Drugs, 27*(2), 135–153.

March, J., Silva, S., Petrycki, S., Curry, J., Wells, K., Fairbank, J., Burns, B., Domino, M., McNulty, S., Vitiello, B., & Severe, J. (2004). Fluoxetine, cognitive-behavioral therapy, and their combination for adolescents with depression: Treatment for Adolescents with Depression Study (TADS) randomized controlled trial. *JAMA, 292*(7), 807–820.

McElroy, S. L., Hudson, J. I., Ferreira-Cornwell, M. C., Radewonuk, J., Whitaker, T., & Gasior, M. (2016). Lisdexamfetamine dimesylate for adults with moderate to severe binge eating disorder: Results of two phase 3 randomized controlled trials. *Neuropsychopharmacology, 41*(5), 1251–1260.

Meltzer, H. Y. (1999). The role of serotonin in antipsychotic drug action. *Neuropsychopharmacology, 21*(2 Suppl.), S106–S115.

Meltzer, H. Y., Alphs, L., Green, A. I., Altamura, A. C., Anand, R., Bertoldi, A., Bourgeois, M., Chouinard, G., Islam, M. Z., Kane, J., Krishnan, R., Lindenmayer, J. P., & Potkin, S. (2003). Clozapine treatment for suicidality in schizophrenia: International Suicide Prevention Trial (InterSePT). *Archives of General Psychiatry, 60*(1), 82–91.

Meltzer-Brody, S., Colquhoun, H., Riesenberg, R., Epperson, C. N., Deligiannidis, K. M., Rubinow, D. R., Li, H., Sankoh, A. J., Clemson, C., Schacterle, A., Jonas, J., & Kanes, S. (2018). Brexanolone injection in postpartum depression: Two multicentre, double-blind, randomised, placebo-controlled, phase 3 trials. *The Lancet, 392*(10152), 1058–1070.

Mostafa, S., Polasek, T. M., Engdahl-Bousman, C., Mueller, D. J., Sheffield, L. J., Rembach, J., & Kirkpatrick, C. M. J. (2022). Pharmacogenomics in psychiatry: The challenge of cytochrome P450 enzyme phenoconversion and solutions to assist precision dosing. *Pharmacogenomics, 23*(16), 857–867.

Nelson, J. C., & Papakostas, G. I. (2009). Atypical antipsychotic augmentation in major depressive disorder: A meta-analysis of placebo-controlled randomized trials. *American Journal of Psychiatry, 166*(9), 980–991.

Nelson, J. C., Baumann, P., Delucchi, K., Joffe, R., & Katona, C. (2014). A systematic review and meta-analysis of lithium augmentation of tricyclic and second generation antidepressants in major depression. *Journal of Affective Disorders, 168*, 269–275.

Nutt, D. J. (2008). Relationship of neurotransmitters to the symptoms of major depressive disorder. *Journal of Clinical Psychiatry, 69*(Suppl. E1), 4–7.

Oslin, D. W., Lynch, K. G., Shih, M. C., Ingram, E. P., Wray, L. O., Chapman, S. R., Kranzler, H. R., Gelernter, J., Pyne, J. M., Stone, A., DeMichele-Sweet, M. A. A., Benitez, J., Becker, M. A., Herbeck Belnap, B., Beizer, J. L., Billups, S. J., Blow, F. C., Chinman, M. J., Coley, K. C., ... Thase, M. E. (2022). Effect of pharmacogenomic testing for drug-gene interactions on medication selection and remission of symptoms in major depressive disorder: The PRIME Care randomized clinical trial. *JAMA, 328*(2), 151–161.

Owen, R., Sikich, L., Marcus, R. N., Corey-Lisle, P., Manos, G., McQuade, R. D., Carson, W. H., & Findling, R. L. (2009). Aripiprazole in the treatment of irritability in children and adolescents with autistic disorder. *Pediatrics, 124*(6), 1533–1540.

Patorno, E., Huybrechts, K. F., Bateman, B. T., Cohen, J. M., Desai, R. J., Mogun, H., Cohen, L. S., & Hernández-Díaz, S. (2017). Lithium use in pregnancy and the risk of cardiac malformations. *New England Journal of Medicine, 376*(23), 2245–2254.

Pittenger, C., Bloch, M. H., & Williams, K. (2011). Glutamate abnormalities in obsessive compulsive disorder: Neurobiology, pathophysiology, and treatment. *Pharmacology & Therapeutics, 132*(3), 314–332.

Posner, K., Brown, G. K., Stanley, B., Brent, D. A., Yershova, K. V., Oquendo, M. A., Currier, G. W., Melvin, G. A., Greenhill, L., Sackeim, H. A., & Mann, J. J. (2011). The Columbia-Suicide Severity Rating Scale: Initial validity and internal consistency findings from three multisite studies with adolescents and adults. *American Journal of Psychiatry, 168*(12), 1266–1277.

Preskorn, S. H. (2013). *Clinical pharmacology of SSRIs*. Professional Communications.

Qaseem, A., Kansagara, D., Forciea, M. A., Cooke, M., & Denberg, T. D. (2016). Management of chronic insomnia disorder in adults: A clinical practice guideline from the American College of Physicians. *Annals of Internal Medicine, 165*(2), 125–133.

Rush, A. J., Trivedi, M. H., Wisniewski, S. R., Nierenberg, A. A., Stewart, J. W., Warden, D., Niederehe, G., Thase, M. E., Lavori, P. W., Lebowitz, B. D., McGrath, P. J., Rosenbaum, J. F., Sackeim, H. A., Kupfer, D. J., Luther, J., & Fava, M. (2006). Acute and longer-term outcomes in depressed outpatients requiring one or several treatment steps: A STAR*D report. *American Journal of Psychiatry, 163*(11), 1905–1917.

Sachs, G. S., Nierenberg, A. A., Calabrese, J. R., Marangell, L. B., Wisniewski, S. R., Gyulai, L., Friedman, E. S., Bowden, C. L., Fossey, M. D., Ostacher, M. J., Ketter, T. A., Patel, J., Hauser, P., Rapport, D., Martinez, J. M., Allen, M. H., Miklowitz, D. J., Otto, M. W., Dennehy, E. B., & Thase, M. E. (2007). Effectiveness of adjunctive antidepressant treatment for bipolar depression. *New England Journal of Medicine, 356*(17), 1711–1722.

Sadock, B. J., Sadock, V. A., & Ruiz, P. (2015). *Kaplan & Sadock's synopsis of psychiatry* (11th ed.). Wolters Kluwer.

Salzman, C. (2005). *Clinical geriatric psychopharmacology* (4th ed.). Lippincott Williams & Wilkins.

Substance Abuse and Mental Health Services Administration. (2024). *Medications for opioid use disorder* (Treatment Improvement Protocol 63). U.S. Department of Health and Human Services.

Sanacora, G., Treccani, G., & Bhagwagar, Z. (2012). Glutamate in the pathophysiology and treatment of mood disorders. *Pharmacological Reviews, 64*(2), 262–298.

Schillinger, D., Piette, J., Grumbach, K., Wang, F., Wilson, C., Daher, C., Leong-Grotz, K., Castro, C., & Bindman, A. B. (2003). Closing the loop: Physician communication with diabetic patients who have low health literacy. *Archives of Internal Medicine, 163*(1), 83–90.

Shapiro, D. A., Renock, S., Arrington, E., Chiodo, L. A., Liu, L. X., Sibley, D. R., Roth, B. L., & Mailman, R. (2003). Aripiprazole, a novel atypical antipsychotic drug with a unique and robust pharmacology. *Neuropsychopharmacology, 28*(8), 1400–1411.

Skapinakis, P., Caldwell, D. M., Hollingworth, W., Bryden, P., Fineberg, N. A., Salkovskis, P., Welton, N. J., Baxter, H., Kessler, D., Churchill, R., & Lewis, G. (2016). Pharmacological and psychotherapeutic interventions for management of obsessive-compulsive disorder in adults: A systematic review and network meta-analysis. *The Lancet Psychiatry, 3*(8), 730–739.

Spitzer, R. L., Kroenke, K., Williams, J. B. W., & Löwe, B. (2006). A brief measure for assessing generalized anxiety disorder: The GAD-7. *Archives of Internal Medicine, 166*(10), 1092–1097.

Stahl, S. M. (2021). *Stahl's essential psychopharmacology: Neuroscientific basis and practical applications* (5th ed.). Cambridge University Press.

Strawn, J. R., Keck, P. E., & Caroff, S. N. (2007). Neuroleptic malignant syndrome. *American Journal of Psychiatry, 164*(6), 870–876.

Tomson, T., Battino, D., Bonizzoni, E., Craig, J., Lindhout, D., Perucca, E., Sabers, A., Thomas, S. V., & Vajda, F. (2018). Comparative risk of major congenital malformations with eight different antiepileptic drugs: A prospective cohort study of the EURAP registry. *The Lancet Neurology, 17*(6), 530–538.

U.S. Food and Drug Administration. (2025). FDA requires expanded labeling about weight loss risk in patients younger than 6 years taking extended-release stimulants for ADHD. U.S. Department of Health and Human Services.

van Dyck, C. H., Swanson, C. J., Aisen, P., Bateman, R. J., Chen, C., Gee, M., Kanekiyo, M., Li, D., Reyderman, L., Cohen, S., Froelich, L., Katayama, S., Sabbagh, M., Vellas, B., Watson, D., Dhadda, S., Irizarry, M., Kramer, L. D., & Iwatsubo, T. (2023). Lecanemab in early Alzheimer's disease. *New England Journal of Medicine, 388*(1), 9–21.

Walkup, J. T., Albano, A. M., Piacentini, J., Birmaher, B., Compton, S. N., Sherrill, J. T., Ginsburg, G. S., Rynn, M. A., McCracken, J., Waslick, B., Iyengar, S., March, J. S., & Kendall, P. C. (2008). Cognitive behavioral therapy, sertraline, or a combination in childhood anxiety. *New England Journal of Medicine, 359*(26), 2753–2766.

Wilson, M. P., Pepper, D., Currier, G. W., Holloman, G. H., Jr., & Feifel, D. (2012). The psychopharmacology of agitation: Consensus statement of the American Association for Emergency Psychiatry Project BETA psychopharmacology workgroup. *Western Journal of Emergency Medicine, 13*(1), 26–34.

Woolf, A. D., Erdman, A. R., Nelson, L. S., Caravati, E. M., Cobaugh, D. J., Booze, L. L., Wax, P. M., Manoguerra, A. S., Scharman, E. J., Olson, K. R., Chyka, P. A., Christianson, G., & Troutman, W. G. (2007). Tricyclic antidepressant poisoning: An evidence-based consensus guideline for out-of-hospital management. *Clinical Toxicology, 45*(3), 203–233.

Yatham, L. N., Kennedy, S. H., Parikh, S. V., Schaffer, A., Bond, D. J., Frey, B. N., Sharma, V., Goldstein, B. I., Rej, S., Beaulieu, S., Alda, M., MacQueen, G., Milev, R. V., Ravindran, A., O'Donovan, C., McIntosh, D., Lam, R. W., Vázquez, G., Kapczinski, F., ... Berk, M. (2018). Canadian Network for Mood and Anxiety Treatments (CANMAT) and International Society for Bipolar Disorders (ISBD) 2018 guidelines for the management of patients with bipolar disorder. *Bipolar Disorders, 20*(2), 97–170.

Zeier, Z., Carpenter, L. L., Kalin, N. H., Rodriguez, C. I., McDonald, W. M., Widge, A. S., & Nemeroff, C. B. (2018). Clinical implementation of pharmacogenetic decision support tools for antidepressant drug prescribing. *American Journal of Psychiatry, 175*(9), 873–886.

www.ingramcontent.com/pod-product-compliance
Lightning Source LLC
LaVergne TN
LVHW052325200926
848481LV00002B/669